Super Nutrition

Get Healthy,
Lose Weight,
Feel Great

Terry McIlroy

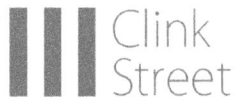

Clink Street

London | New York

Published by Clink Street Publishing 2019
Copyright © 2019

First edition.
The author asserts the moral right under the Copyright, Designs and Patents Act 1988 to be identified as the
author of this work.

ISBN: 978-1-913136-08-6
ebook: 978-1-912562-67-1

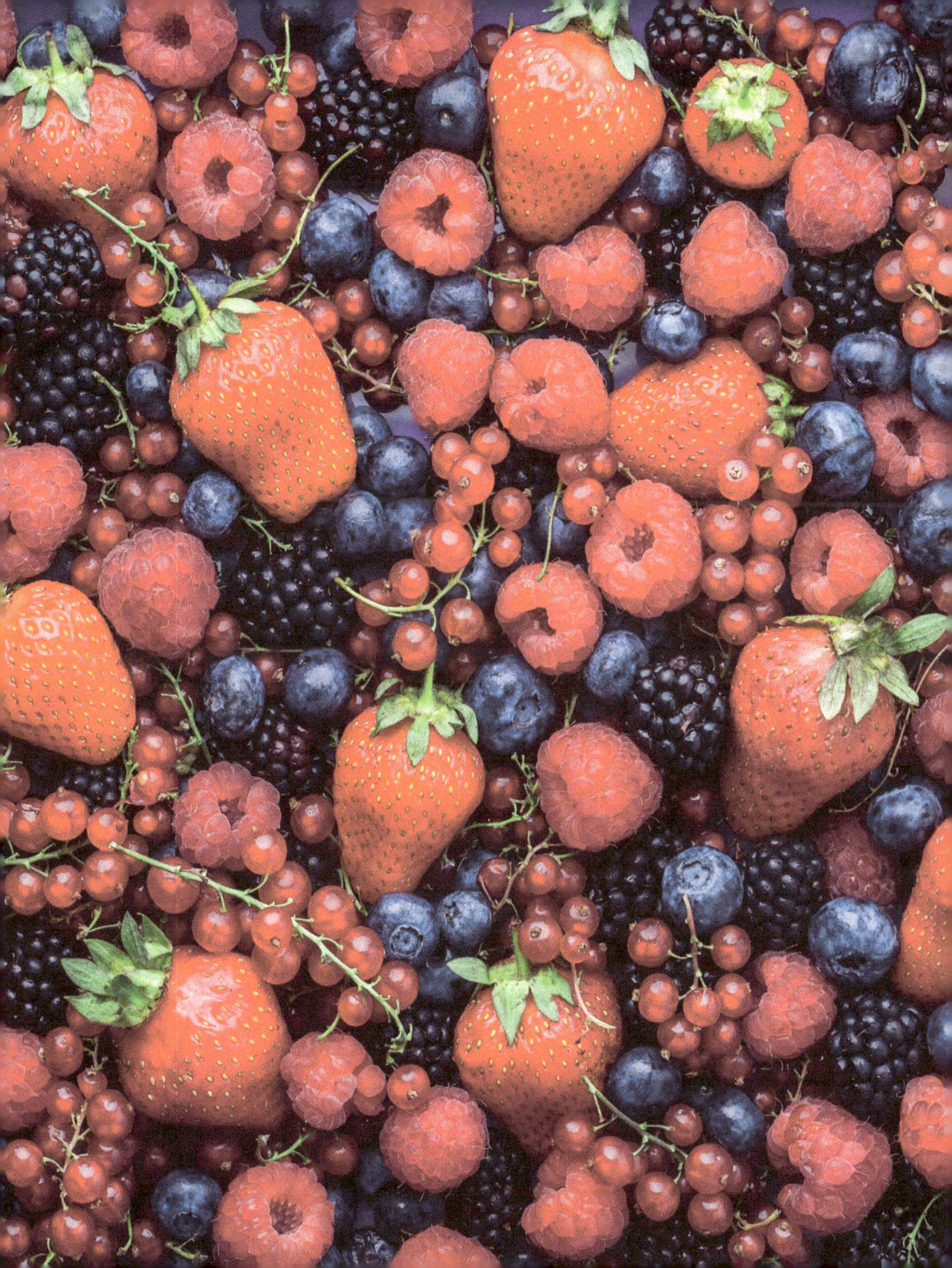

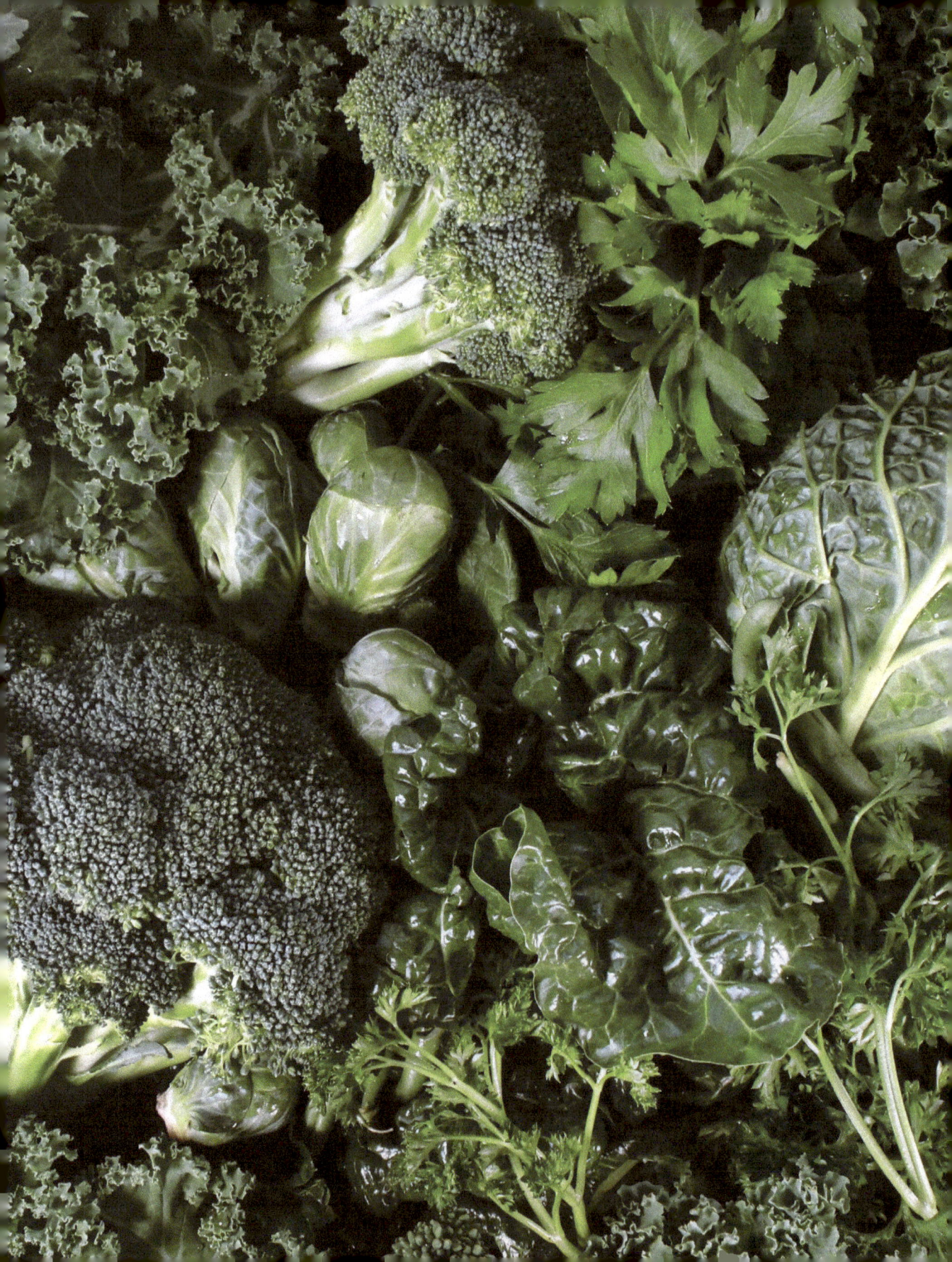

CONTENTS

DEDICATION   IX
INTRODUCTION   XI
WHAT IS THIS BOOK ABOUT?   XIII
EQUIPMENT YOU WILL NEED (OTHER THAN THE NORM)   XIV
MY TOP TEN HEALTH TIPS   XVI
ORGANIC! WHAT DOES IT MEAN?   XIX
EMBRACE EPSOM SALTS   XXI
SALT OF THE EARTH   XXIII
APPLE CIDER VINEGAR   XXV
SWEETEN WITH RAW LOCAL NATURAL HONEY   XXVII

THE RECIPES   1

RISE AND SHINE WITH FRESH JUICES AND SCENTED INFUSIONS   3
BREAK THE FAST   23
SUPER SMOOTHIES   43
SERIOUS SALADS   65
SOUPS DE JOUR   85
OUR DAILY BREAD   108
LUSH LUNCHES   121
HEALTHY SNACKS   141
PROPER DINNERS   161

EXAMPLE WEEKLY MEAL PLANNER   180
MY WEEKLY MEAL PLANNER   181

ACKNOWLEDGEMENTS   183
DISCLAIMER   183

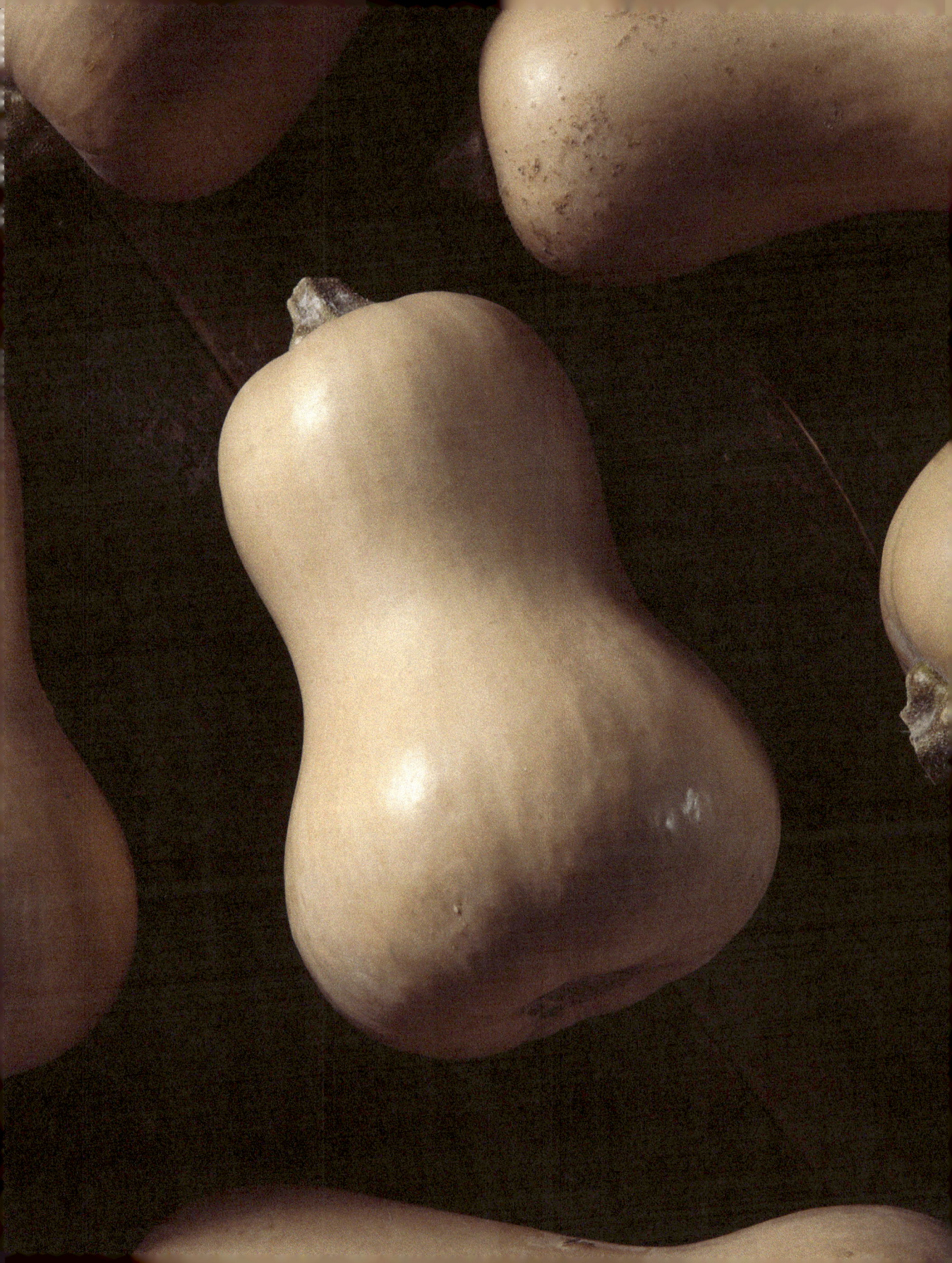

This is real wholesome healthy food to nourish your body, mind and spirit

TERRY MCILROY

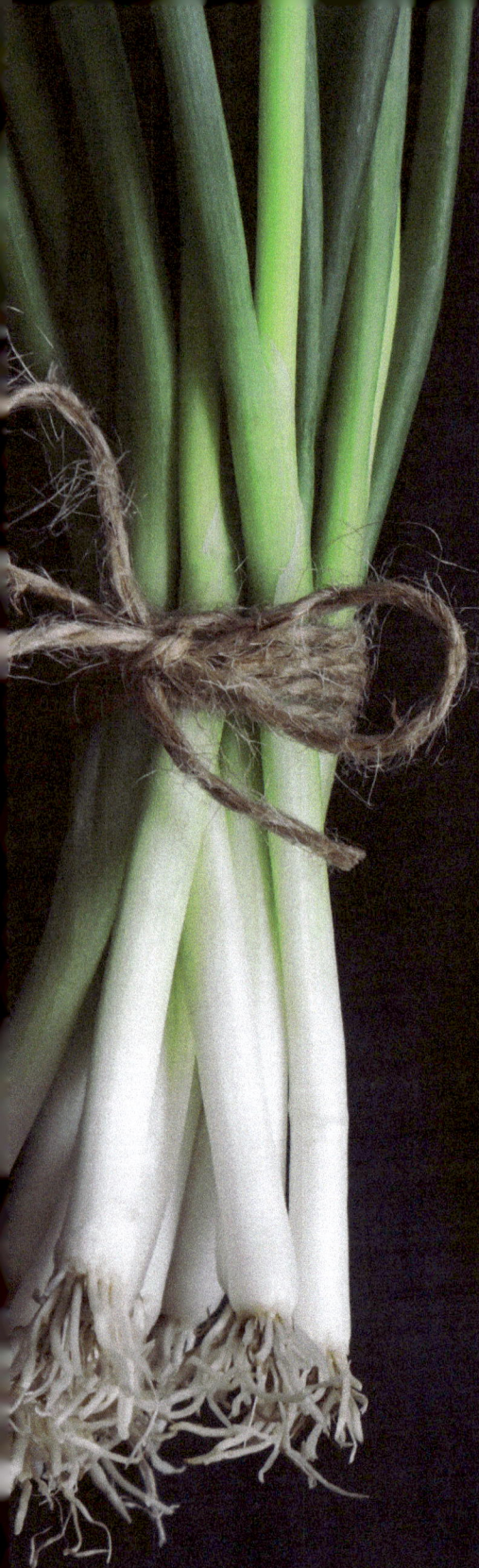

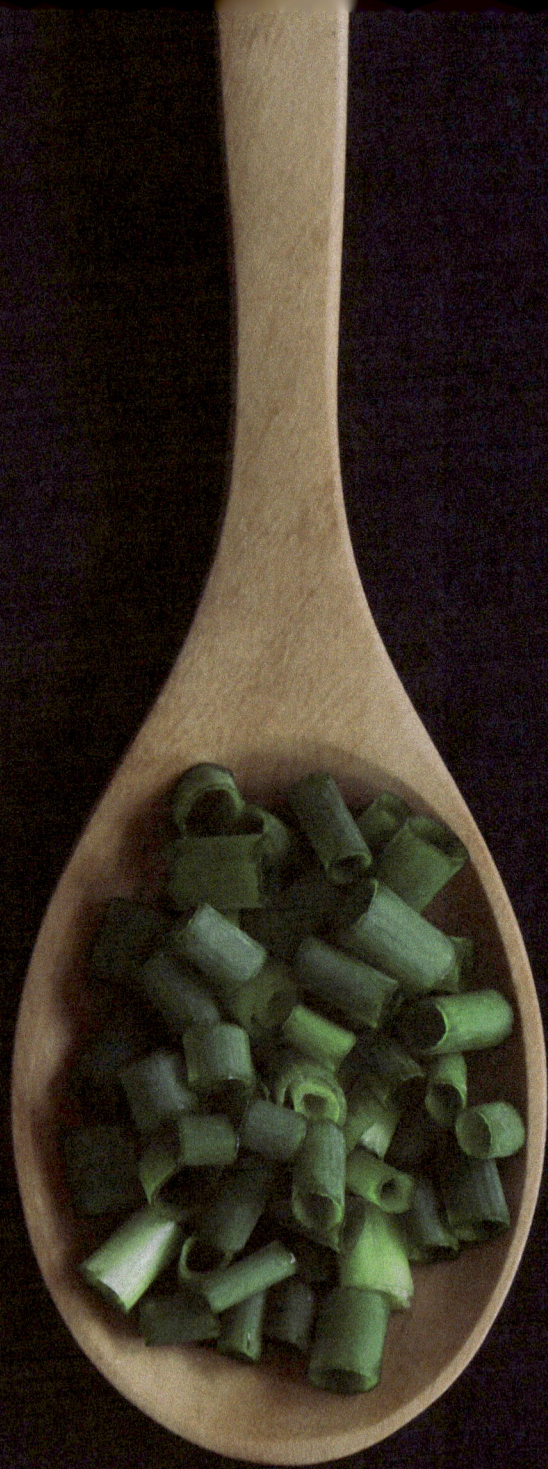

DEDICATION

As a young teenager, I couldn't wait to get out and work, in order to earn my own money to buy the things I wanted. My auntie told me that a local guesthouse that she worked in, were looking for staff to do the dishes, I didn't hang about, I contacted Rayanne House (Guesthouse and fine dine restaurant in Holywood, Co. Down) about the vacancy and after meeting Anne McClelland (proprietor) I was given the chance to start. I began by doing the dishes and some cleaning duties, however after meeting Raymond McClelland and his son Connor, who were the main chefs, I quickly became fascinated, observing the beautifully presented food that they were producing for their prestige guests. After about six months Raymond and Anne took me under their wing and introduced me to the world of catering and hospitality, teaching me all their unique recipes and techniques, ranging from their outstanding personalised breakfast dishes and menus, through to patisserie, starters, sorbets, ice-creams, salads and eventually main courses, all of which were in keeping with the classical French-style cuisine. Connor decided to move to America to open up his own restaurant (which was very successful) and so I became Raymond's prodigy. I tortured him with questions every minute I spent with him, because I wanted to learn so much from him as he was one of the country's leading and well respected chefs, winning a plethora of awards throughout his career. As time went on I became more and more competent, so I decided to go to college and get my cooking qualifications. Raymond and Anne provided me with chef whites and knives and I quickly received my certificates. After about five years with Rayanne, I decided to leave, and I went on to have a fairly successful cheffing career, with many ups and downs.

Unfortunately Raymond passed away a couple of years after I left, which was a massive shock and loss for the family and me too, as he was my mentor.

I would like to dedicate this book to the late Raymond McClelland, because I would not be the creative, imaginative and passionate chef I am today, had it not been for the time he invested in me, sharing his vast knowledge and training

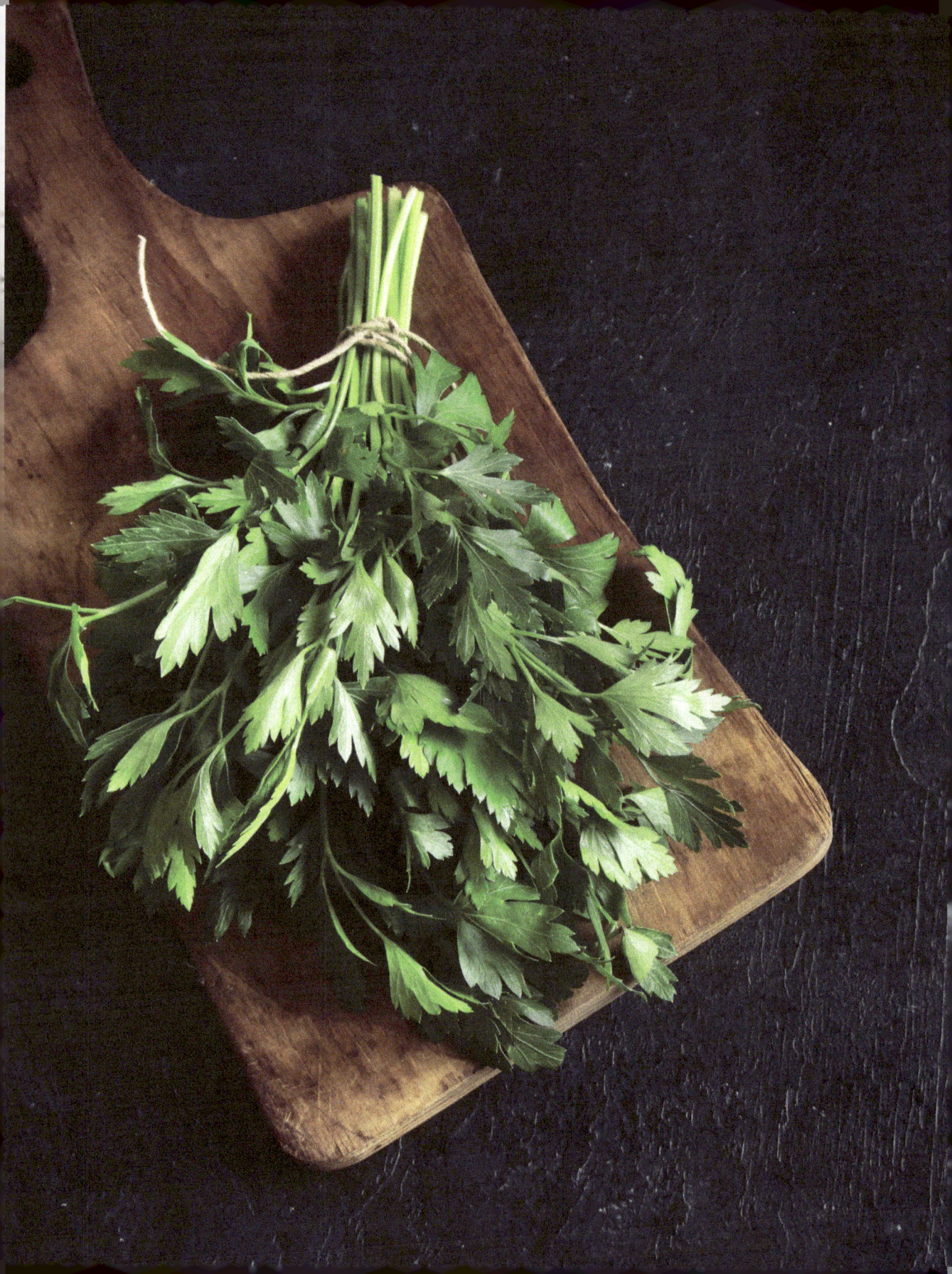

INTRODUCTION

First things first, let me say thank you for purchasing my book. I'm confident that you will get great value from it, even if you only make some of the recipes – use the rest for inspiration to create your own balanced meals, and get on the right path of good health and happiness.

All my life, I have been plagued with severe acne and constant mouth ulcers. The obvious protocol was to go to the doctor, so I did, hundreds of times. I was prescribed all sorts of drugs, Roaccutane for acne to steroids for the ulcers in my mouth, to name but a few, and the side effects were worse than the problem they were meant to be treating – nose bleeds, flaking skin, puffiness, etc. I was then referred to many different specialists, with ultimately no success whatsoever in alleviating my issues. Later in life, it became clear to me that pharmaceuticals were not working for me personally, and this is when I started asking myself the question "What is causing my health problems?" My thought process shifted to 'cause and effect' and I wondered if maybe, just maybe, what if what I was eating, or more importantly not eating, could be the cause, and the presenting symptoms were the effect?

I started to get very interested in health and nutrition, so I bought a juicer and a smoothie machine and started consuming more fruits and vegetables. I also went to see a nutritionist, who suggested reducing or eliminating dairy products for a while. Lo and behold, just by making these small dietary adjustments, cutting out fizzy drinks and drinking lots of pure water, my presenting symptoms were all but gone after a period of three to four weeks, no mouth ulcers or acne for the first time in my life! Eureka!

I was now convinced that sound nutrition is vital for good health! However I knew deep down that my experience was just the tip of the iceberg and I wanted to learn more.

So I enrolled on a three-year part-time nutrition diploma course with the College of Naturopathic Medicine in Belfast. Going back to school essentially was quite daunting, however I was hungry for the knowledge, and it was at the midpoint of the course, when I decided that I wanted to combine my skills as a chef with my newfound passion 'nutrition' and start creating my own recipe book. After receiving my official qualification in October 2017, I started spending every spare minute I had creating the recipes that follow.

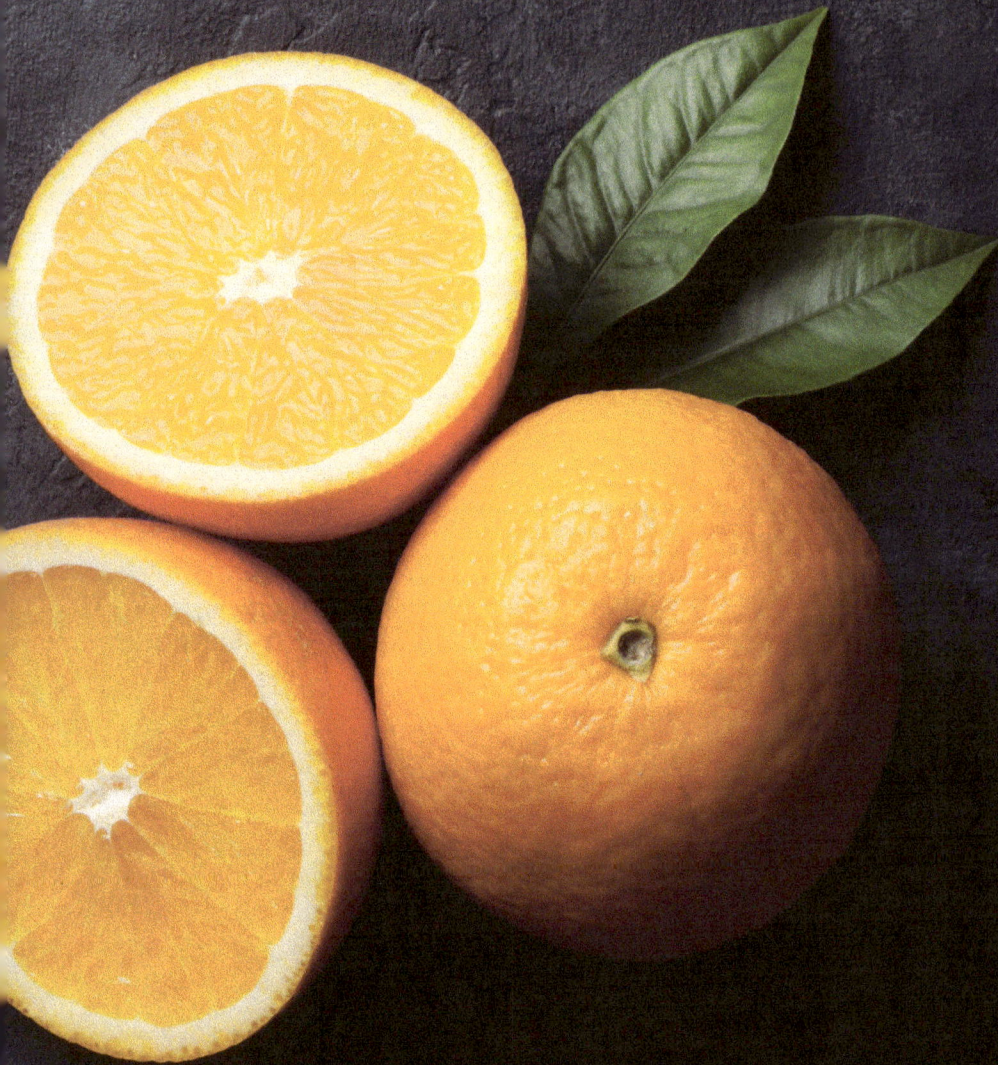

WHAT IS THIS BOOK ABOUT?

This book is a complete eating plan, in which you can design your daily menus to work around your busy lifestyle. The main focus is on natural detoxification and ensuring the consumption of a full spectrum of macronutrients (protein, complex carbs and good fats) and micronutrients (vitamins, minerals and phytonutrients) over the period of any given week. Nourishing your body on a cellular level. I believe in nutrients not calories! We have natural feedback systems within us that maintain balance (homeostasis). It is vital to our health that we stay in a state of equilibrium. When balance is disrupted, we may be at risk of illness – reasons for this can be, poor diet, lack of exercise, smoking, drug abuse, exposure to toxins, high stress, etc. which can all lead to disease causing inflammation. Informed nutrition and lifestyle choices help us stay in homeostasis.

My recipes are all constructed with a therapeutic aim at the foundation, and built into satisfying, delicious meals and drinks which will make you feel great whilst consuming them, and you will be motivated and inspired to try more and more as you journey through from front to back. You will look forward to making each dish, as I have done all the hard graft to give you the confidence in knowing your meals are not just delicious, they are nutritionally balanced.

Who can benefit from this book?

Well everyone really, there is great variety to suit all dietary models. It is also a great tool for nutritional therapists, and the one healthy recipe book everyone has to have. Completely unique recipes to cater for all tastes, this is your one stop shop for any healthy meal or beverage, everyday!

EQUIPMENT YOU WILL NEED
(OTHER THAN THE NORM)

- teapot diffuser
- ice-cube trays (4)
- slow masticating juicer
- electric citrus juicer
- nutri-bullet (or better)
- handheld stick blender
- food processor
- food mixer with dough hook
- a good set of sharp knives
- stainless steel pots
- non-stick frying pans (chemical free)
- measuring cups
- measuring spoons
- actifry/air fryer
- slow cooker

- ziplock bags
- glass jars with clasp lids
- non-stick traybake tray 32cm x 22 cm
- wire rack
- 9 cm stainless steel cooking rings x 4
- non-stick silicone mat
- spatula
- pestle & mortar
- grater
- large piping bag with fluted nozzle
- stainless steel baking tray 20cm x 26cm x 5 cm
- chopping boards

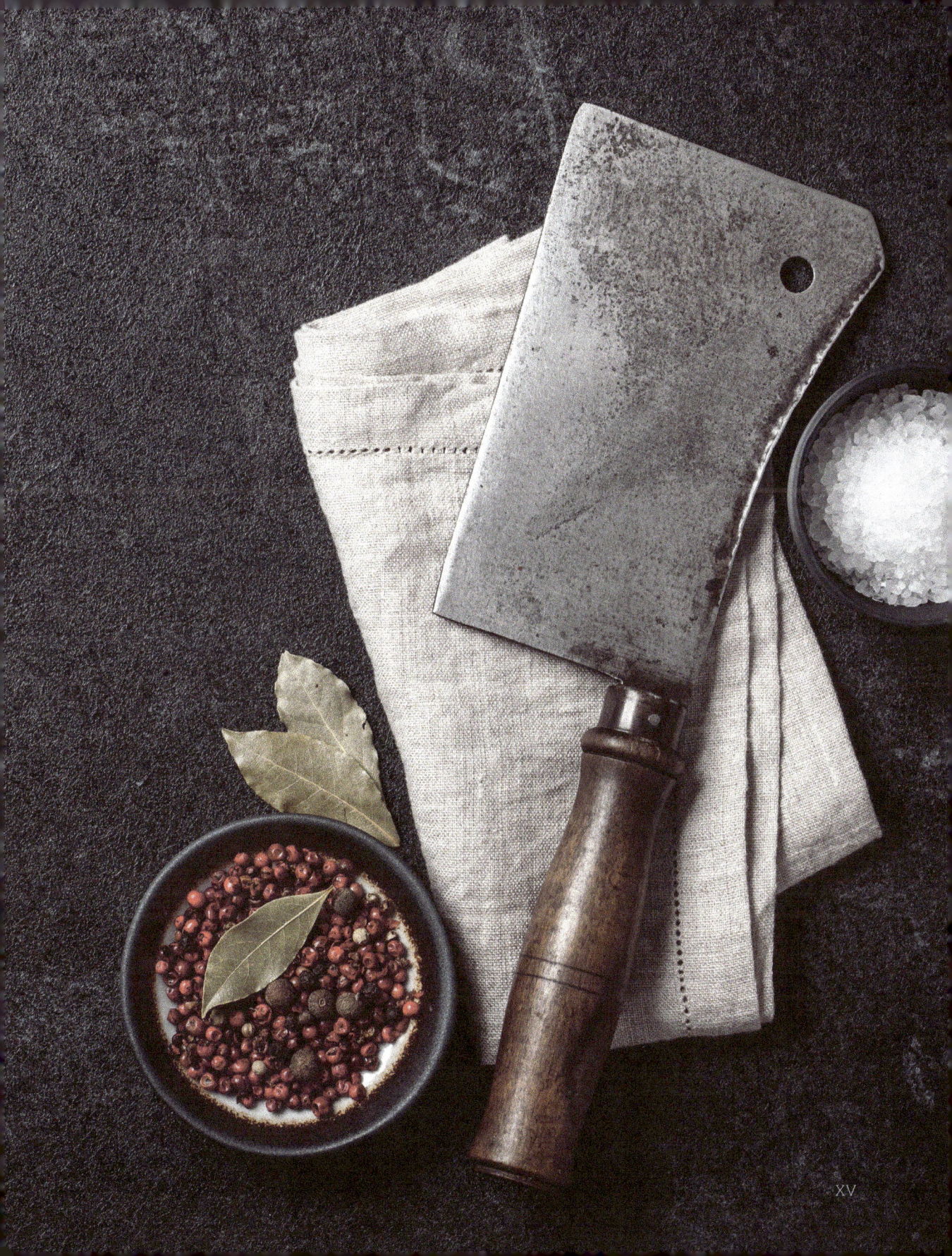

MY TOP TEN HEALTH TIPS

1

Choose organic produce (including toiletries & cosmetics) when possible, to reduce your toxic load. Non-organic fruit and veg can be washed in water and a little apple cider vinegar to lower the chemical levels

2

Reduce caffeine & eliminate fizzy drinks, Drink 2–3 litres of filtered water daily for adequate hydration (herbal teas count towards this)

3

Take 1 gram of high quality vitamin C supplement daily

4

Take Regular exercise, including weight-bearing exercise (doctor permitting!!) & PRACTICE A FORM OF MEDITATION (yoga combines the two)

5

Ensure you are getting adequate unbroken sleep, 7–8 hours every night, if not, try to determine the cause and correct it

6

Avoid all processed foods & refined sugar, consume more raw vegetables and fruit

7

Get out in the sunshine (when it appears) and practice deep breathing in the fresh air to boost vitamin D and oxygen levels

8

Focus on nutrients not calories, eat the rainbow

9

Look after your teeth and gums with good dental hygiene practice

10

If you smoke, please QUIT! & Have a positive mental attitude

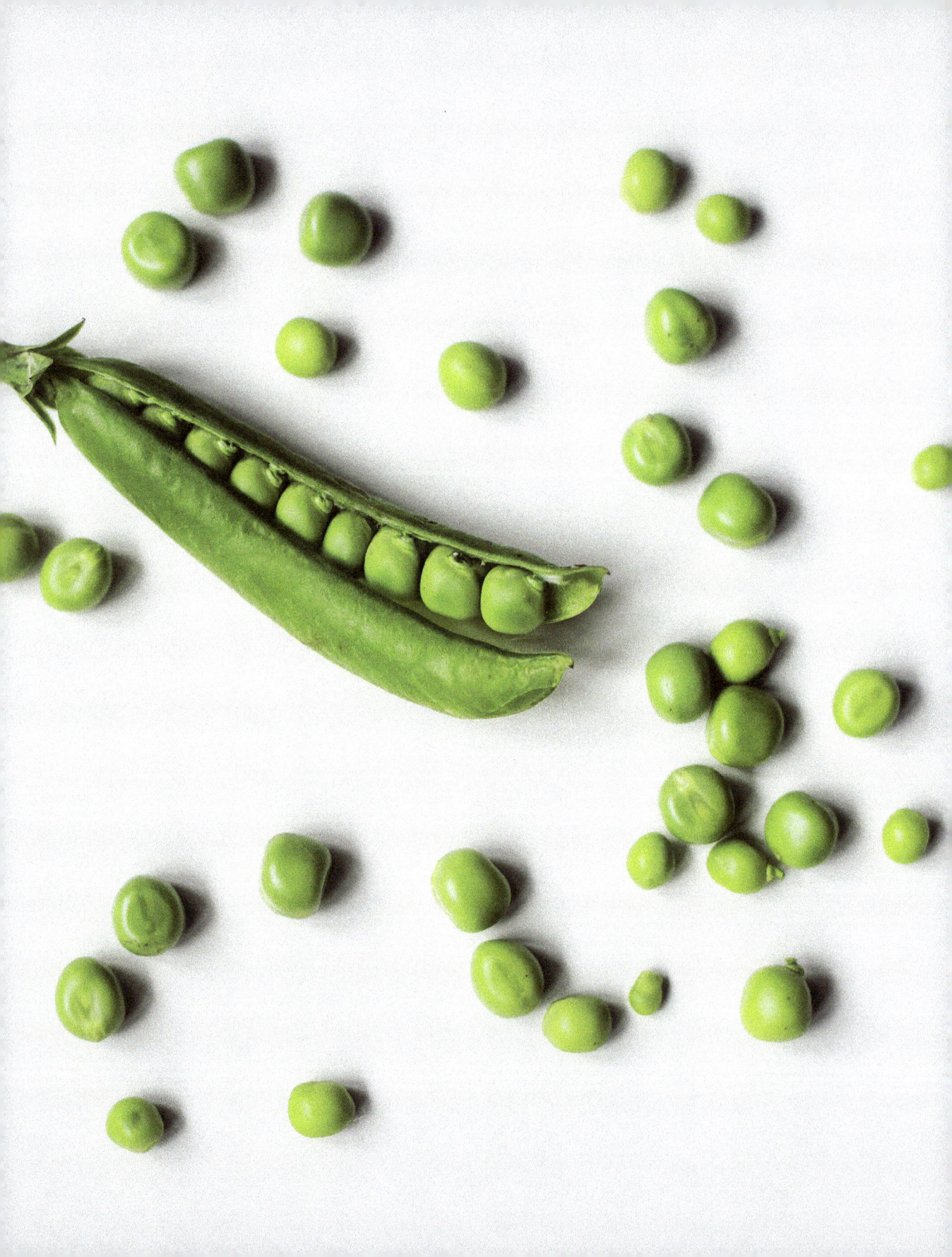

ORGANIC! WHAT DOES IT MEAN?

.

Organic food is free from fertilisers, pesticides, growth regulators, additives, preservatives and weed killers.

.

Organic food legislation prohibits the use of Genetically Modified Organisms (GMO's)

.

Organic food has significantly more vitamins, minerals and nutrients than conventional.

.

Organic is a return to tradition when food was produced naturally, as it should be.

.

Obviously it will not always be possible to solely purchase organic food due to financial reasons, however every time we do we are voting with our money to increase demand. Try to source local organic farmers and markets, buy direct from them for more competitive prices.

.

Research the 'Dirty Dozen and the Clean Fifteen' to help you make better choices when buying fruits and vegetables

.

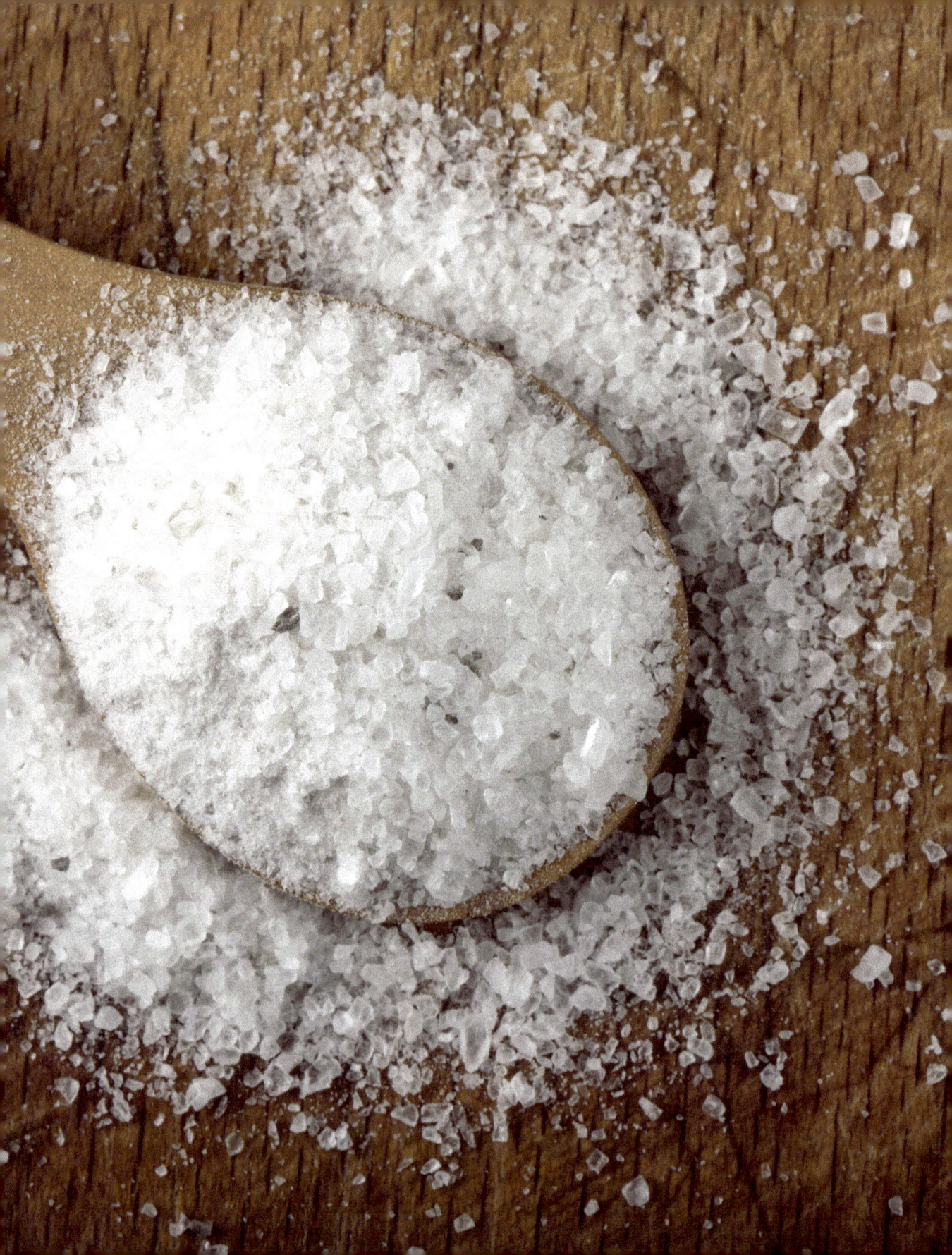

EMBRACE EPSOM SALTS

•

Epsom salts are packed with magnesium (the anti-stress mineral) which is absorbed through your skin when you have an Epsom salt bath.

•

Magnesium is fundamental to the normal function of hundreds of bodily functions, including, muscle & nerve stimulation, oxygenation, circulation and the regulation of inflammation.

•

Epsom salts baths support and encourage the natural detoxification process by extracting toxins out from the body via the skin.

•

Epsom salts baths restore minerals and have demonstrated pain relief in muscles and joints.

•

Pregnant women or people with obvious skin issues (cuts, burns, scrapes etc.) should avoid Epsom salts baths. Always consult your doctor if you have any health conditions before taking an Epsom salts bath.

•

Directions for drawing an Epsom salts bath.

Fill your tub to the desired level, ensuring the water is not too hot and at a comfortable temperature. Pour in 500 grams approx. of Epsom salts, swish the water around to help dissolve and disperse the salts.

Try to stay in the bath for 40 minutes in order to take maximum advantage of the health benefits it offers, do this 2-3 times per week.

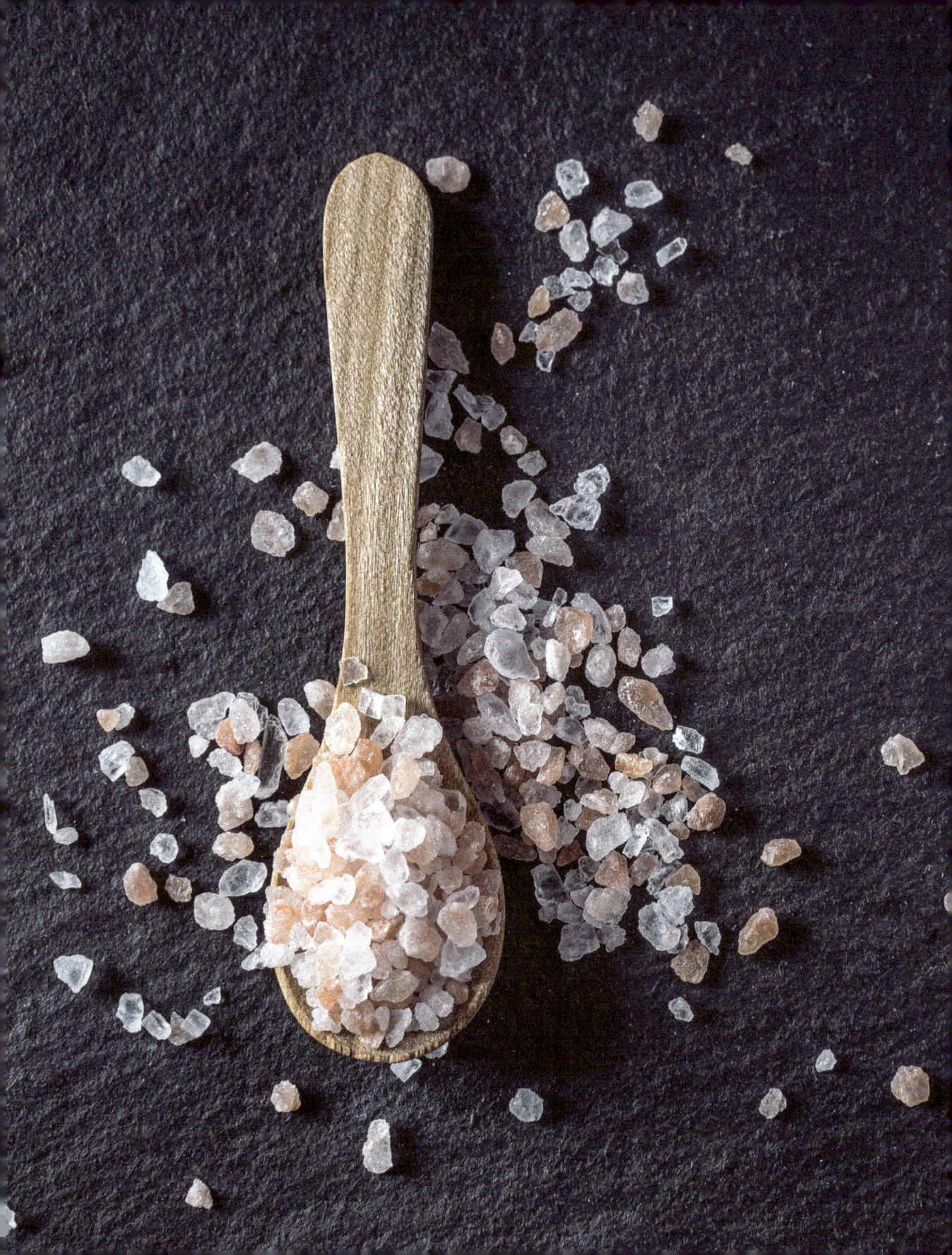

SALT OF THE EARTH

•

Pink Himalayan Salt contains 84 trace minerals including, Potassium, Magnesium, Iron, Calcium & Sodium, which are all essential to the body for various functions, ranging from preventing dehydration, regulating blood pressure to energy production.

•

Pink Himalayan Salt is a potent detoxifier. When added to water it transforms into an ionic solution that supports the withdrawal of toxins via the skin and fat tissues.

•

Pink Himalayan Salt helps to improve digestion and increase satiety and also boosts blood sugar health.

•

Pink Himalayan Salt helps prevent muscle cramps, regulates sleep, supports libido, improves bone strength, supports respiratory & vascular health and promotes healthy ph balance on a cellular level.

Regular table salt is a heavily processed, unnatural, chemically cleaned refined product, which is stripped of all of its minerals, making it 99% sodium chloride, furthermore, anti-caking agents are added to make it easier to pour. Sodium is fundamental for survival, however it needs the other minerals to work synergistically within us.

Time to switch?

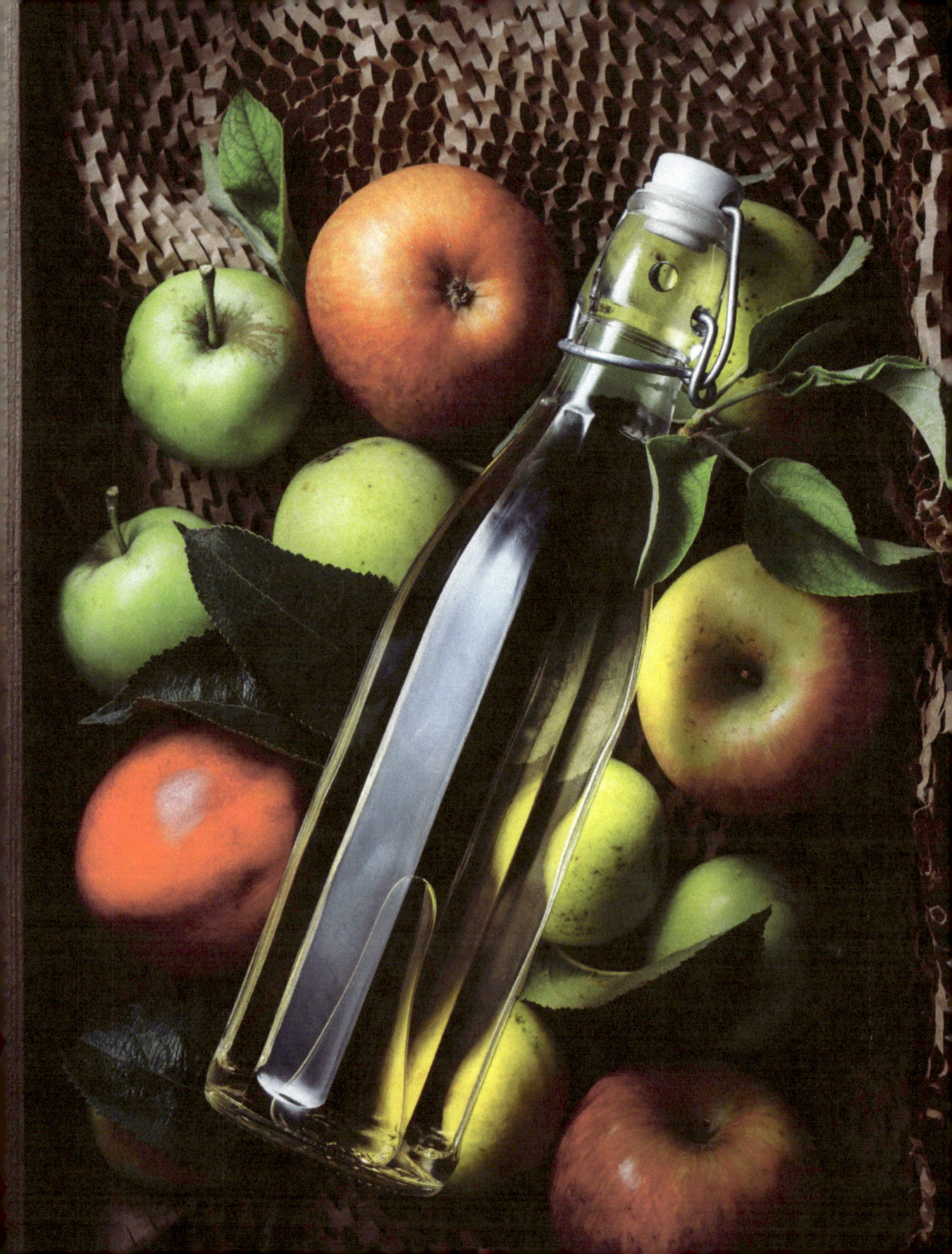

APPLE CIDER VINEGAR

Choose Organic, Raw, Unfiltered Apple Cider Vinegar (with the mother) To gain these health benefits

- Rich in enzymes & potassium
- Support a healthy immune system
- Helps control weight
- Promotes digestion & ph Balance
- Helps soothe dry throats
- Promotes natural detoxification
- Regulates blood sugar
- Lowers Cholesterol
- Improves skin health
- Reduces blood pressure
- Relieves symptoms of acid reflux
- Boosts beneficial gut bacteria

add a couple of capfuls of acv to a glass of warm water and some raw organic honey, for a refreshing elixir.

Use as a condiment and in cooking for a tangier flavour than white or malt vinegar.

ACV can be used topically on the skin to treat sunburn, fungus and even varicose veins.

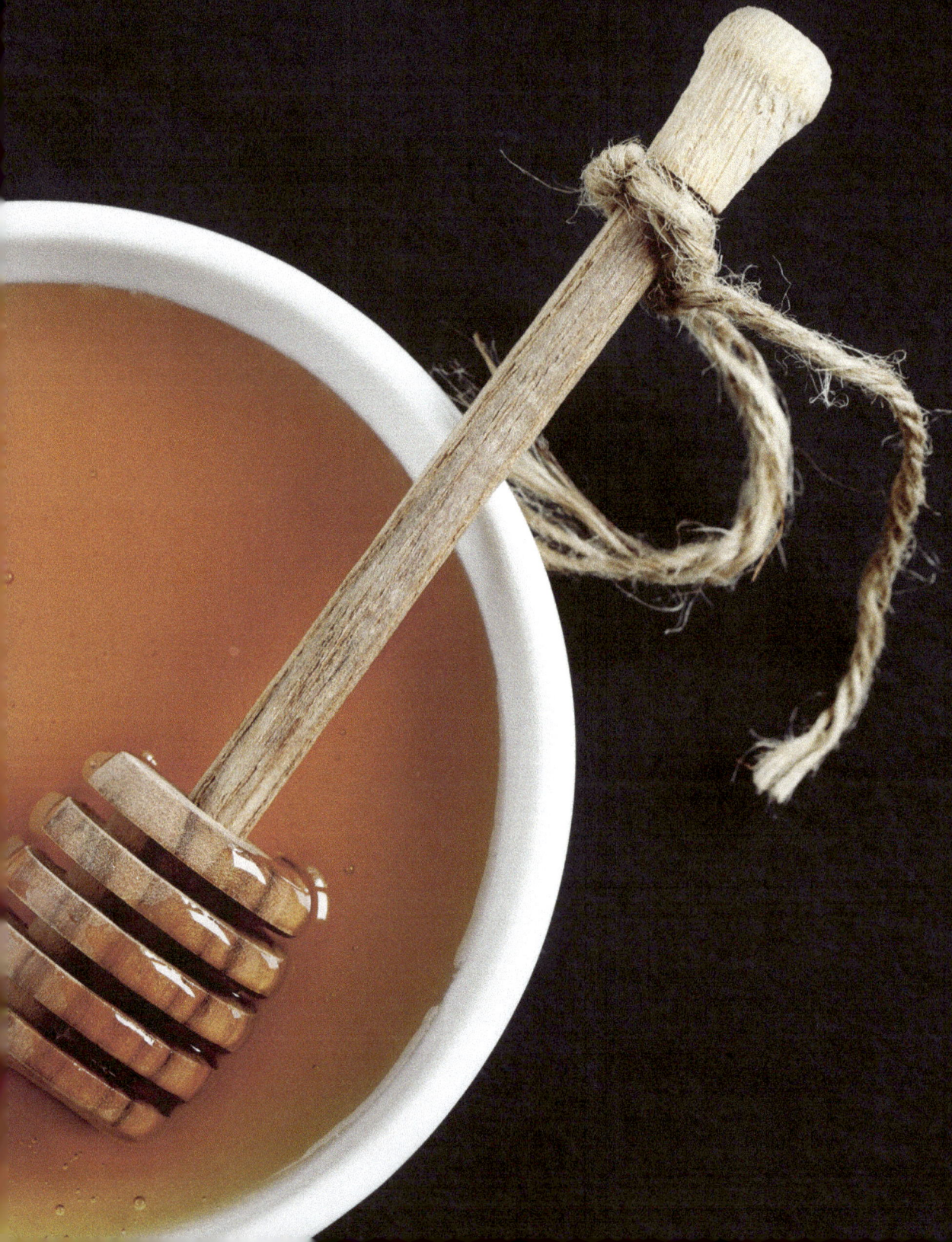

SWEETEN WITH RAW LOCAL
NATURAL HONEY

Raw honey is an Anti-oxidant Powerhouse, which boosts your immune system, helping you fend off disease.

Raw honey has Anti-bacterial, Anti-viral and Anti-fungal properties.

Raw Honey is the perfect energy source for your liver.

Raw honey is packed with amino acids, nutrients, minerals and live enzymes, in contrast, conventional honey is refined, heat treated and devoid of health benefits.

Raw honey benefits sleep, digestion, skin health, blood sugar health and cholesterol levels.

Raw honey contains Bee Pollen (natures complete food), perfectly balanced with carbohydrates, Fats, Protein, vitamins and minerals.

Raw honey may not be suitable for people with allergies. Always consult your doctor if you have any health concerns before switching to raw honey. Raw honey is not suitable for children.

THE IMPORTANCE OF PLANNING
AND PREPARATION

Prep like a pro, plan your weekly meals and allocate time to do your shopping and 'mise en place' (French for making sure all preparation is done before you begin cooking)

Planning and preparation are your keys to success, use the weekly meal planner on page 180 which you can photocopy to construct your individual personalised menus.

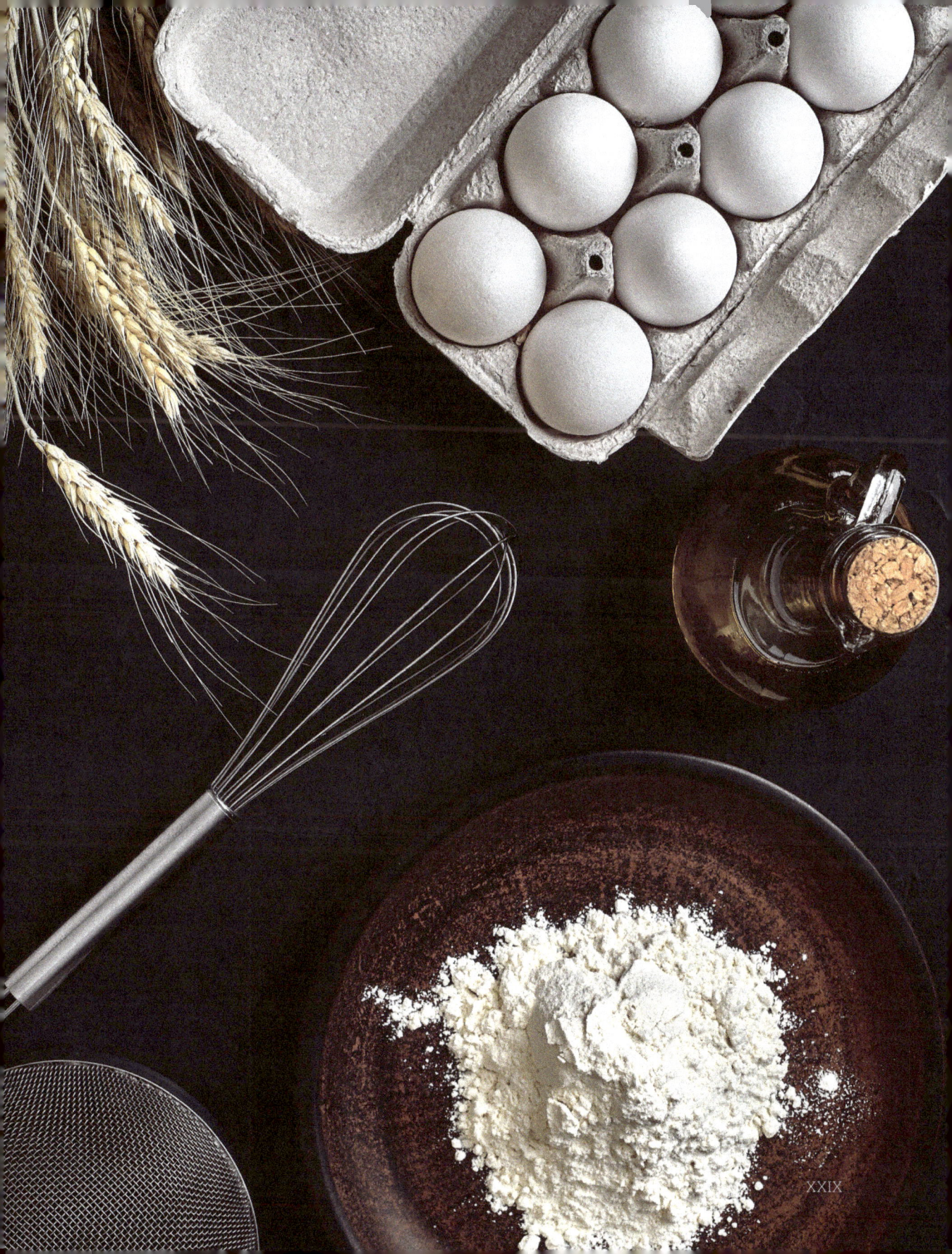

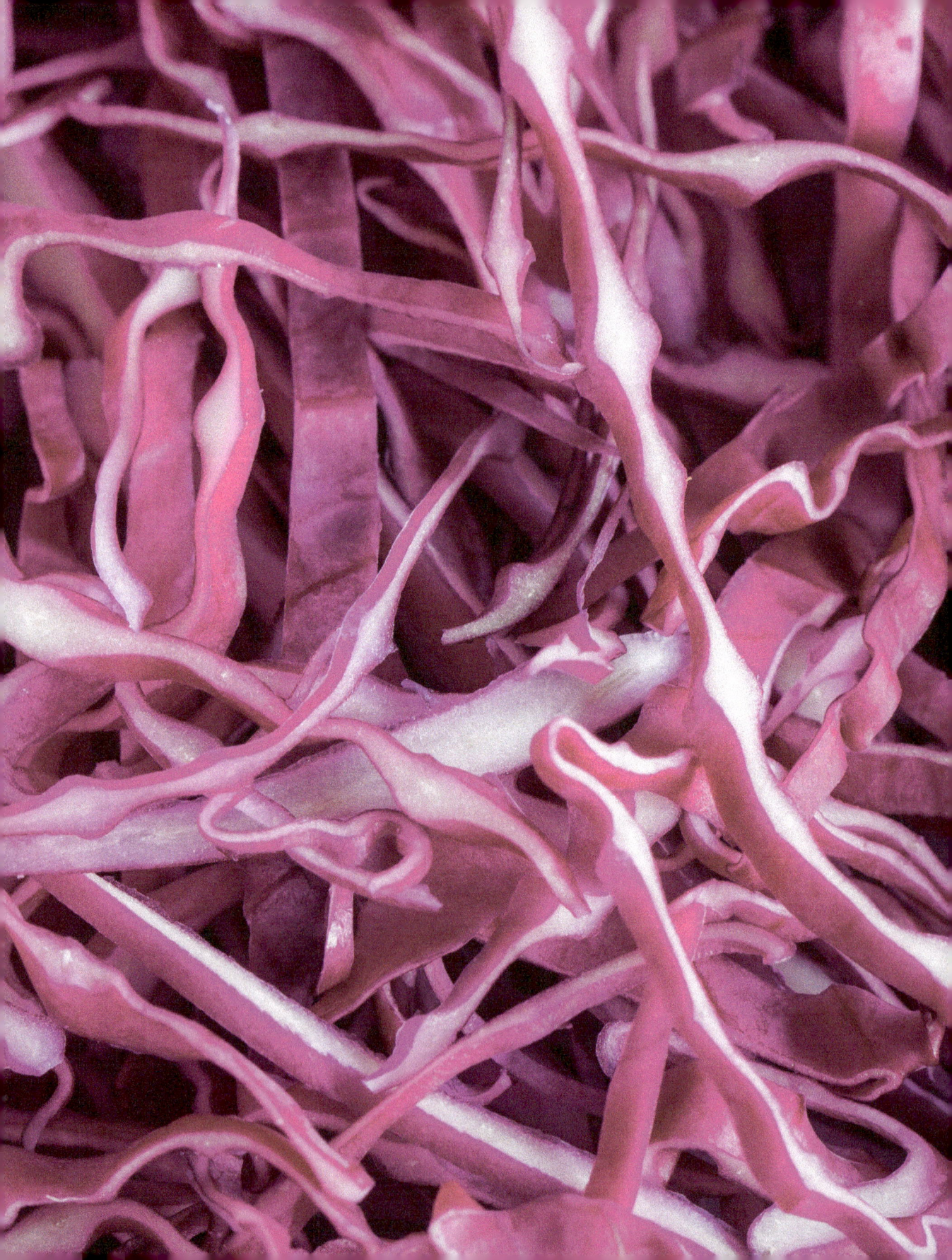

GET
HEALTHY

LOSE
WEIGHT

FEEL
GREAT

♡

THE RECIPES

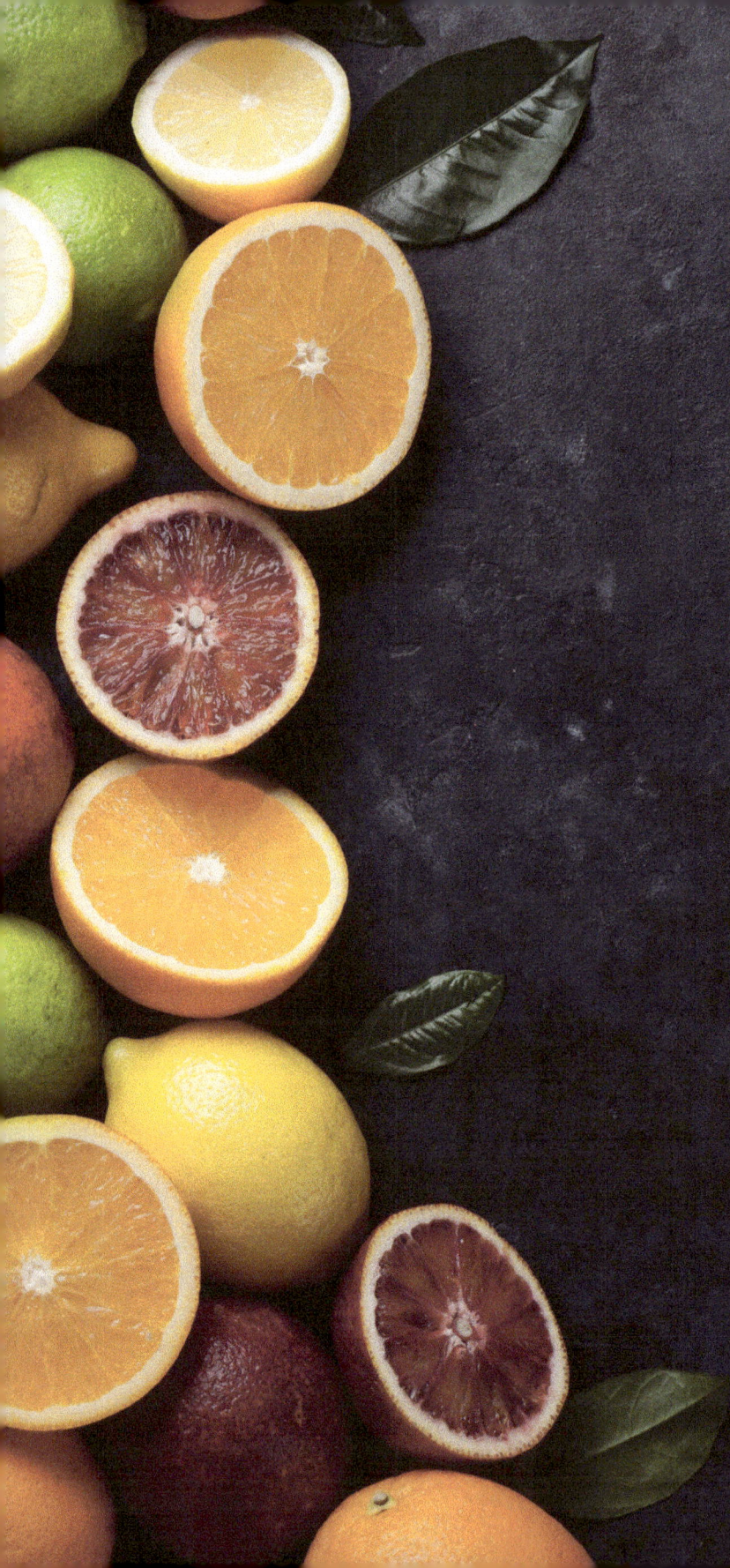

RISE AND SHINE WITH FRESH JUICES AND SCENTED INFUSIONS

Whilst the beverages in this chapter can be enjoyed any time of the day, they are best taken upon waking from a restful sleep, which supports the natural process of detoxification and elimination, delivering micronutrients and hydration to your cells.

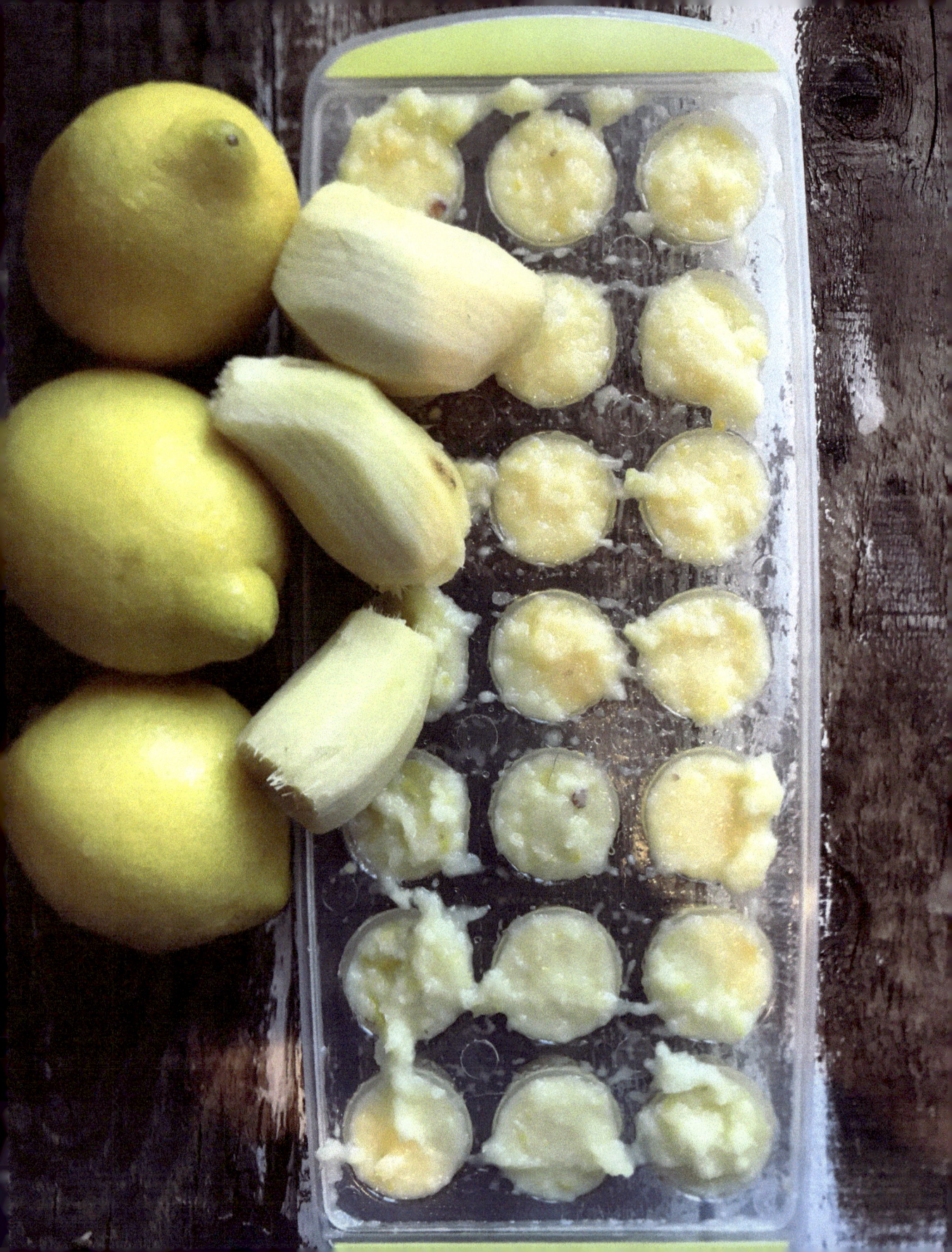

LEMON & GINGER
FROZEN CUBES

MAKES APPROX. 40 CUBES

5 unwaxed, organic Lemons

500 grams fresh ginger

100 mls water

4 ice cube trays

Wash lemons and roughly chop (peel, pith & flesh, the lot!)

Peel and roughly chop the ginger

Place ingredients in a food processor, blitz for 1 min, stop and scrape down the sides, blitz again pouring in the water for approx 3 mins, or until you have achieved a fairly smooth consistency.

Spoon the mixture into your ice cube trays, Freeze for at least 6 hours.

Remove cubes from trays and place in a zip-lock freezer bag & keep in the freezer for handy use.

Place 2–3 cubes in a teapot infuser and fill with boiling water, stir and allow to infuse for 5 minutes before enjoying.

They are also a great addition to your smoothies.

Lemon is excellent for detoxification as well as being alkalising, and Ginger has powerful anti-inflammatory properties.

CITRUS DANDELION TEA

SERVES 1 – 2

½ Lime, ½ Lemon & ½ Orange,
all unwaxed

1 organic dandelion root teabag

500mls–1000mls approx of boiling water

Adjust water and fruit content to suit your taste.

Slice citrus fruits and place in a tea infuser or a cup or glass of your choice along with the dandelion root teabag.

Boil water and let stand for 1 minute, then pour over the ingredients, stir and leave for 5 minutes before enjoying.

Dandelion and citrus fruits support healthy liver function, boosts immunity and promotes healthy skin.

MINTED GREEN TEA

SERVES 1 – 2

2 Large sprigs of fresh mint

1 Green teabag

1 Peppermint teabag

500mls – 1000mls approx. of boiling water

Adjust water content to suit your taste.

Place Mint & Teabags in a tea infuser or cup or glass of your choice.

Boil water and let stand for 1 minute, then pour over ingredients, stir and leave for 5 minutes before enjoying.

Green Tea is high in Antioxidants and Mint relieves indigestion.

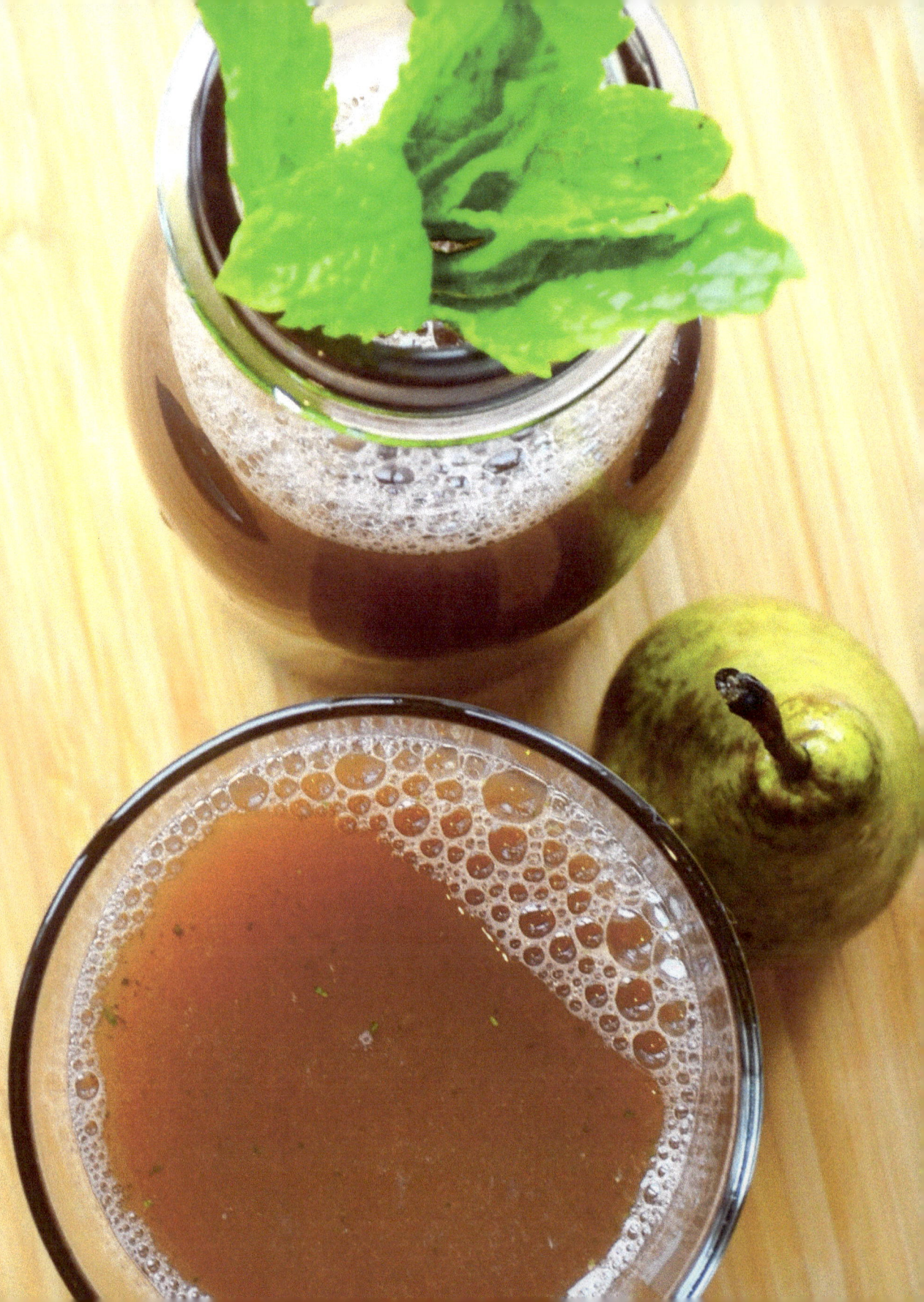

PEAR, CUCUMBER, WATERMELON & MINT COOLER

SERVES 2

½ Watermelon

2 Conference pears

½ Cucumber

1 Handful of fresh mint

I use a slow masticating juicer for most of my juice recipes, because I believe it delivers a much superior tasting juice with less foam, whilst preserving vital nutrients.

Peel the watermelon and chop into pieces that will fit the shoot of your juicer.

Wash and chop the cucumber, pears and mint.

Place the sieve in the collection receptacle.

Start this juice with the mint to ensure maximum nutrient extraction from the herb, followed by the cucumber, pears and watermelon.

This cool juice is very hydrating, excellent for aiding digestion and can be enjoyed at any time of the day.

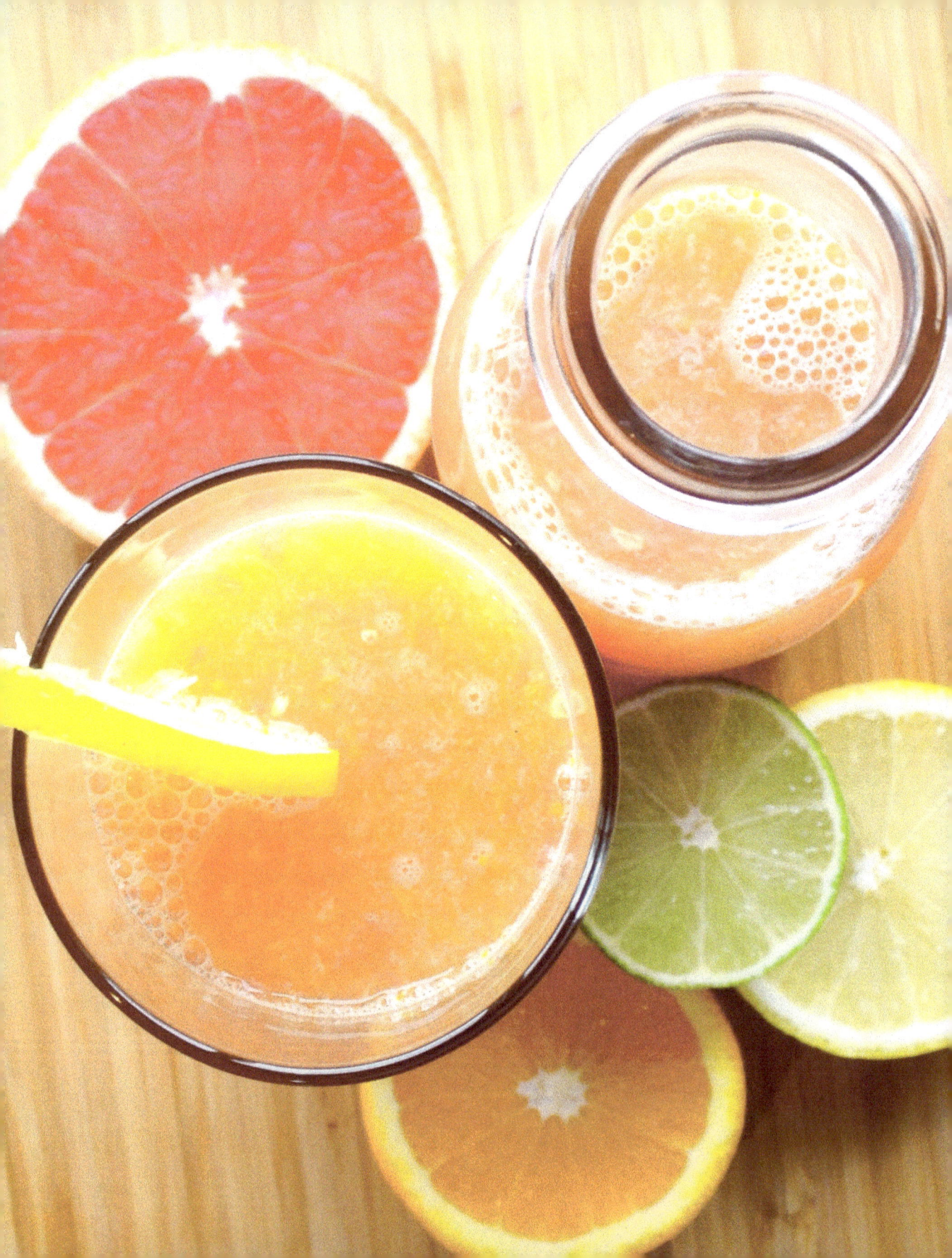

CITRUS DETOX

SERVES 2

3 Large juicy oranges

1 Ruby or red grapefruit

1 Lime

1 Lemon

The electric citrus juicer is the best, most efficient method to extract the bounty of nutrients from these citrus fruits.

Cut all the citrus fruits (across the equator) so to speak.

Juice in any order.

You will need to use a small glass or container to collect the juice, which will need to be transferred 3 to 4 times to a larger glass/container for stirring, this ensures an even taste and colour.

Stir well and enjoy.

A great way to get your vitamin C first thing in the morning.

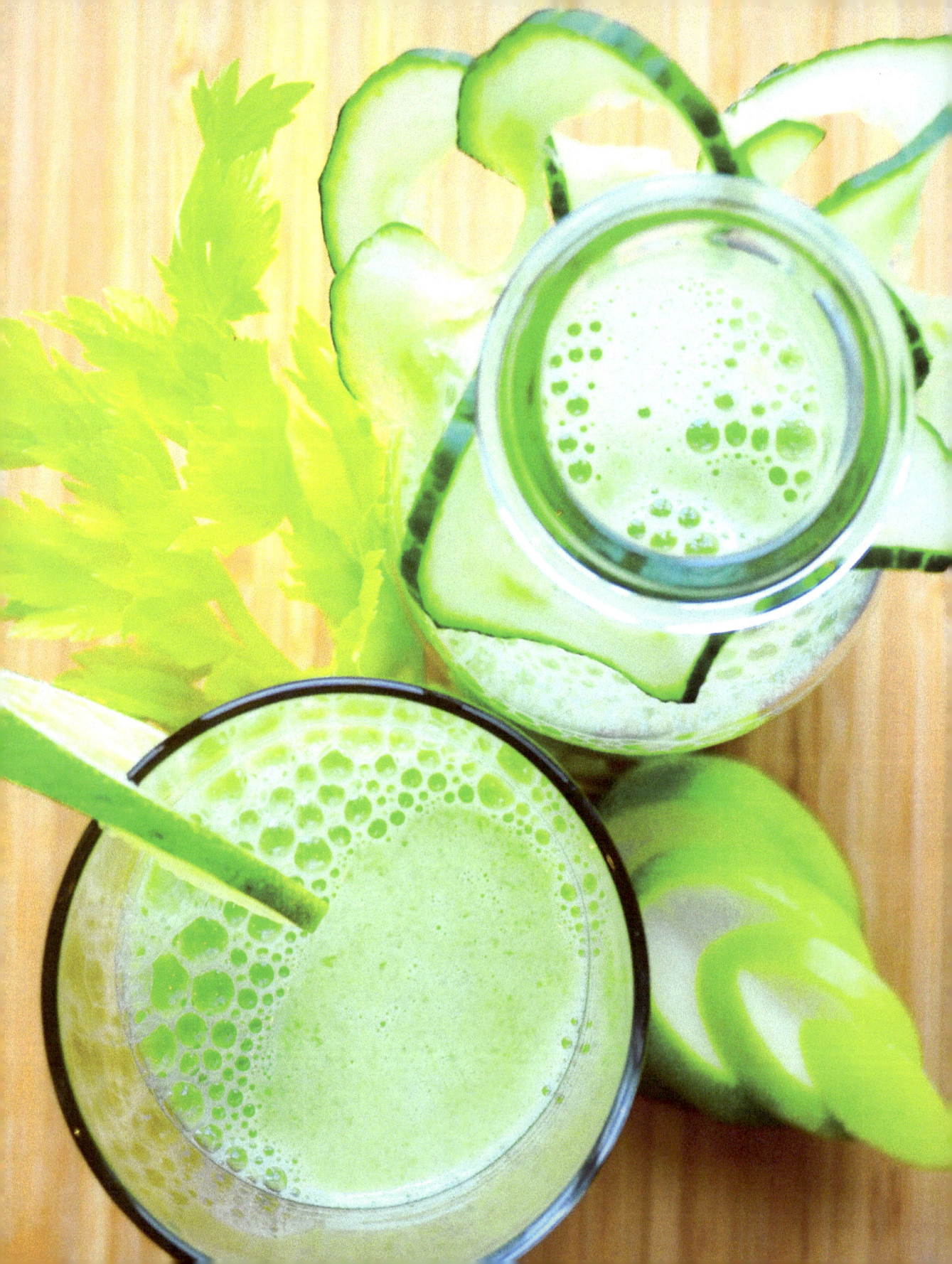

GRANNY SMITH APPLE, CELERY, CUCUMBER, ACV AND LIME

SERVES 2

3 Granny smith apples

2 Celery ribs

½ Lime

½ Cucumber

1 Tbsp Apple cider vinegar (with the mother)

50 Mls filtered water (approx)

Wash, core and chop apples into small pieces to fit the shoot of your juicer.

Wash and chop the celery, cucumber & lime in the same fashion.

Juice all the ingredients with the sieve in place and stir in the apple cider vinegar.

Taste the juice, if it's too sharp for you, dilute with some water.

'An apple a day keeps the doctor away' A source of pectin, a water soluble fibre which supports digestive health and promotes healthy cholesterol levels.

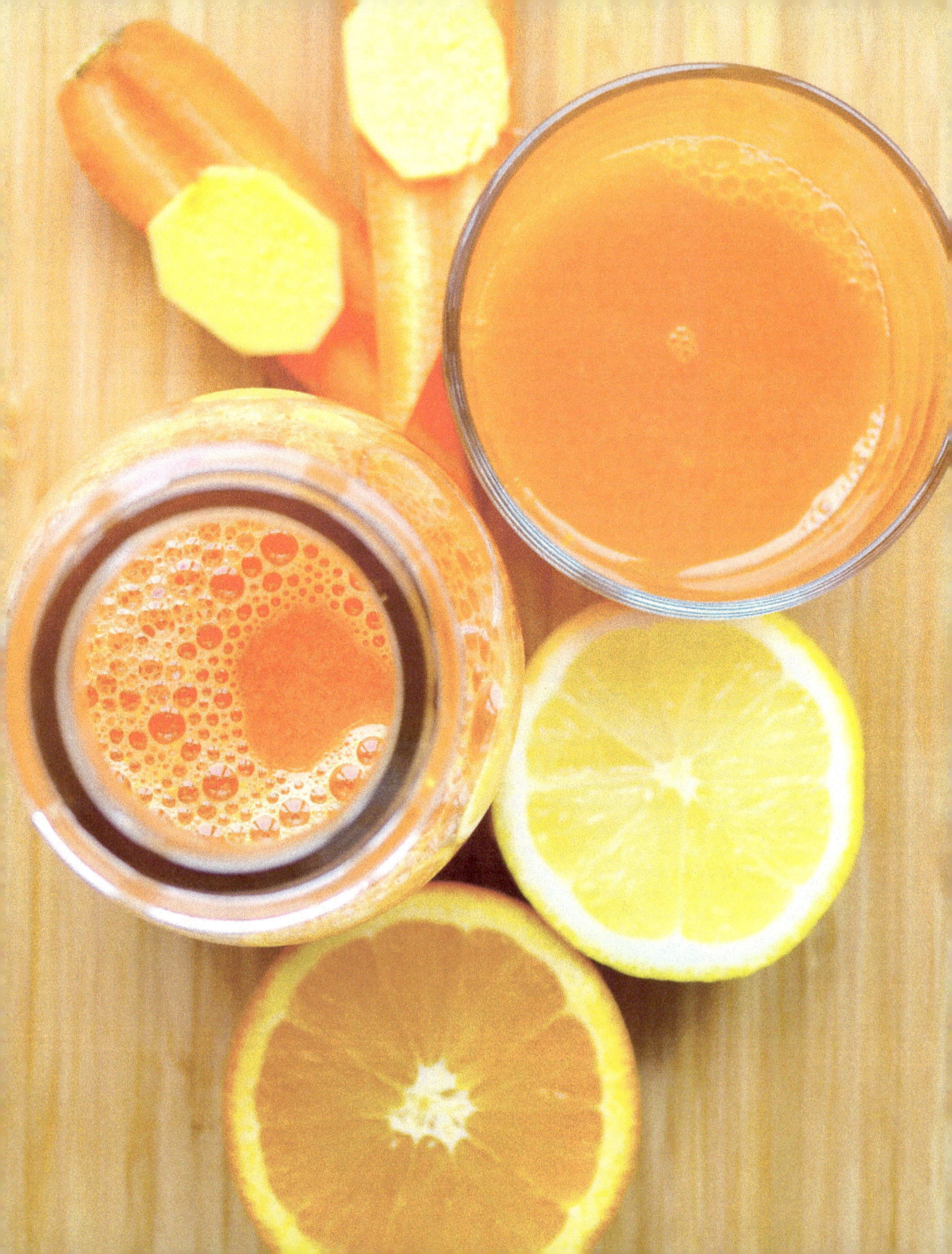

SUNSHINE SHERBET SURPRISE

SERVES 2

2 Oranges

½ Lemon

4 Medium carrots

1 Thumb-size piece of ginger

Peel, chop and wash carrots to fit shoot of your juicer.

Peel and chop ginger

Cut oranges and lemon in half.

Juice the carrots and ginger in the slow masticating juicer with the sieve in place.

Juice the oranges and lemon using the electric citrus press, pour through the sieve and mix with the carrot and ginger.

Mix and serve.

Keep your eyesight tiptop with this delicious Zingy Juice full of beta carotene & vitamin C

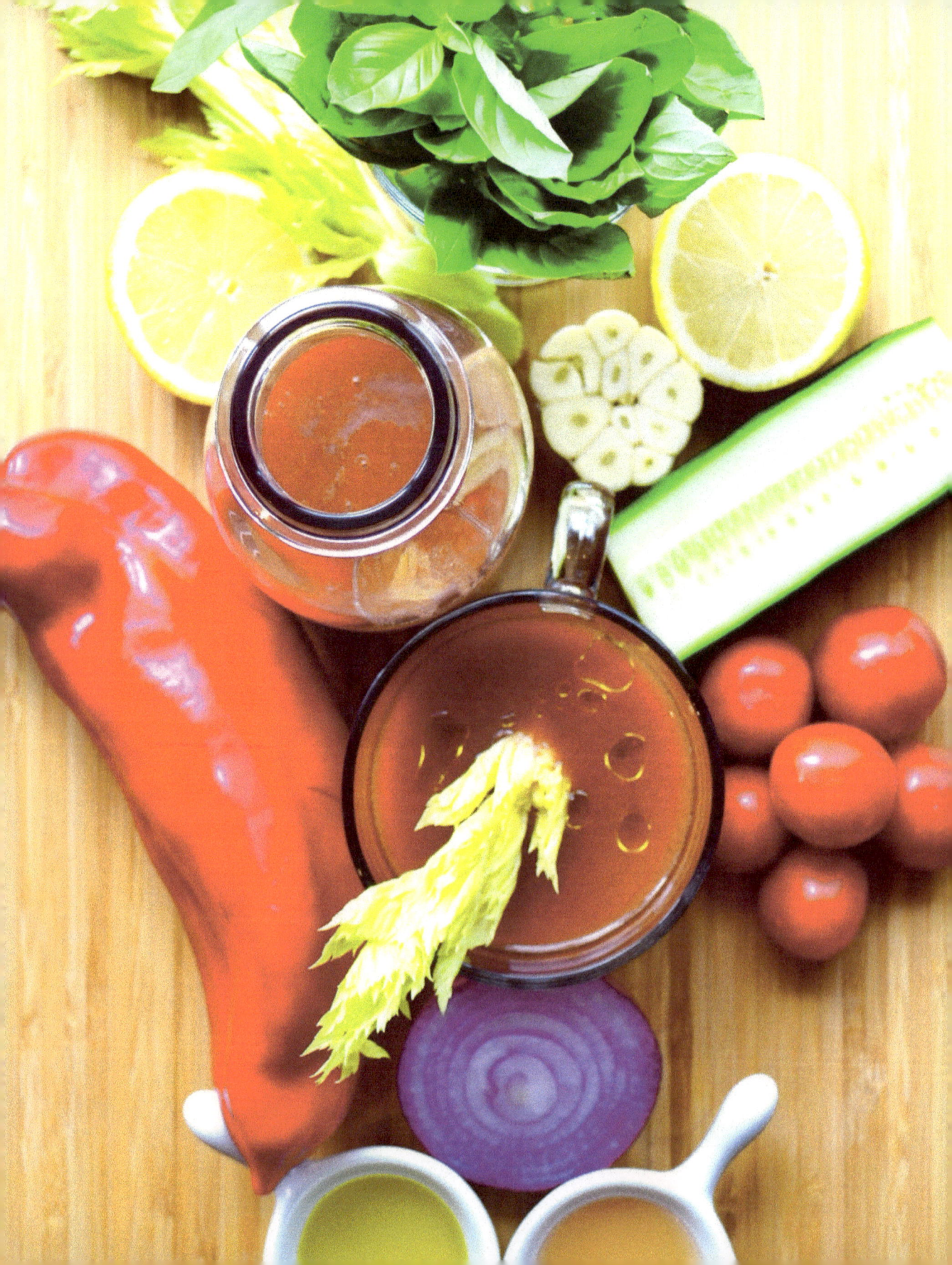

BLOODY MARY GAZPACHO

750 grams Sweet plum cherry tomatoes

1 Rib of celery

1 Pointy sweet red pepper

1 Clove of garlic

½ Cucumber

¼ Red onion

4 Sprigs of basil

¼ Lemon

10 mls Apple cider vinegar (with the mother)

Dash of Worcestershire sauce (contains anchovy)

Dash of Tabasco sauce

2 tbsp organic extra virgin olive oil

A pinch of Himalayan pink salt

This juice can clog up the small sieve that is usually supplied with your slow juicer, therefore it is best to pass all the liquid after the recipe is complete with a larger sieve, whisk and bowl.

Wash & chop celery, pepper, cucumber, red onion and basil to fit the shoot of your juicer.

Wash tomatoes and juice all of the ingredients.

Add Worcestershire sauce, ACV, Tabasco sauce & salt.

Whisk and pass through a fine sieve, stir in olive oil.

Tomatoes and Red peppers are a great source of the antioxidant Lycopene, which has many health benefits including reducing risk of heart disease and cancer (in particular prostate cancer in men).

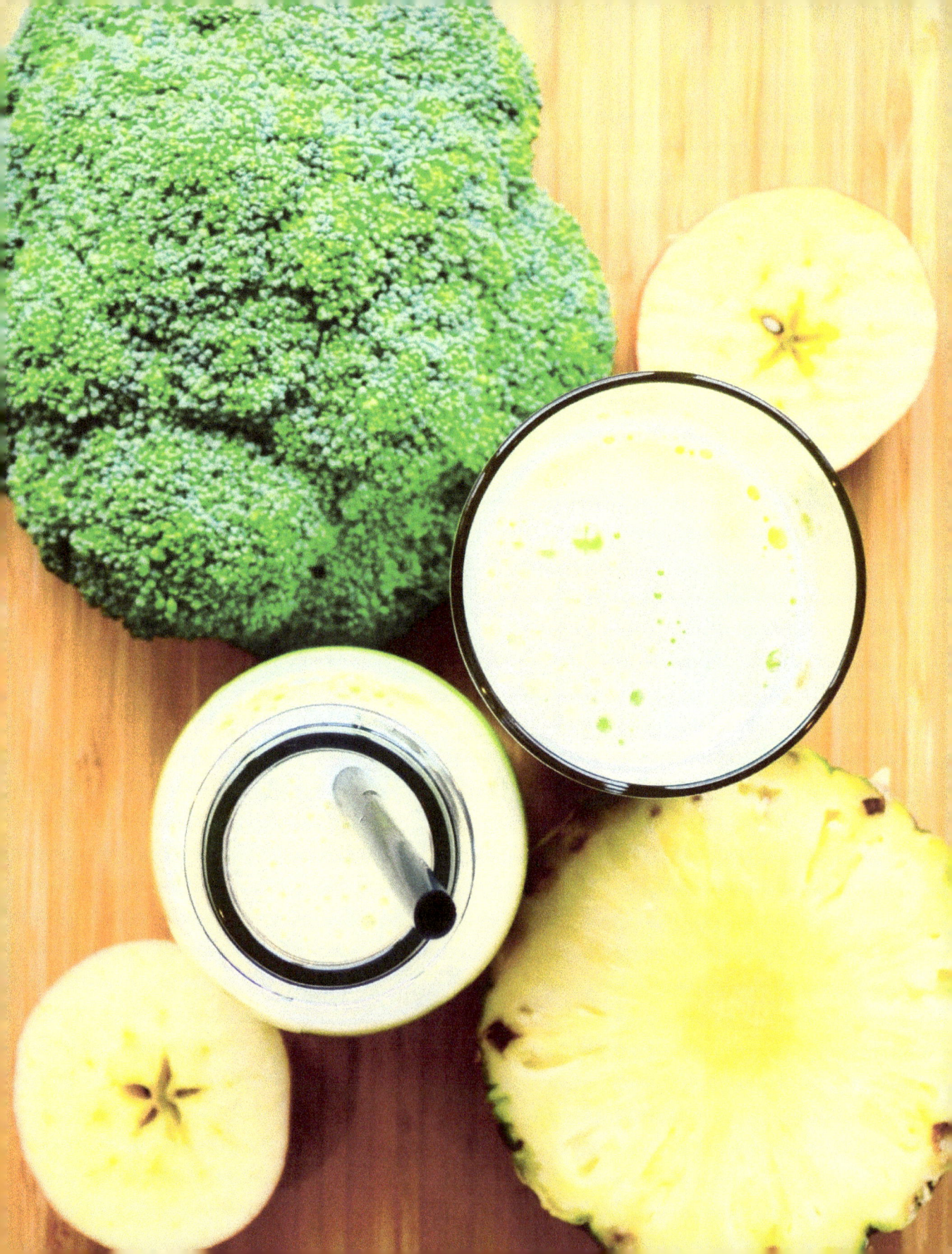

APPLE, BROCCOLI & PINEAPPLE

SERVES 2

2 Royal gala apples

½ Pineapple

½ Head of broccoli

Wash, core and chop apples into small pieces.

Wash and chop broccoli.

Peel and chop pineapple. (don't remove core)

Juice the ingredients through the slow juicer with the sieve in place.

Stir and enjoy.

Pineapple contains an enzyme called bromelain, which is concentrated in the core. Bromelain is an powerful anti-inflammatory compound and also a great digestive aid.

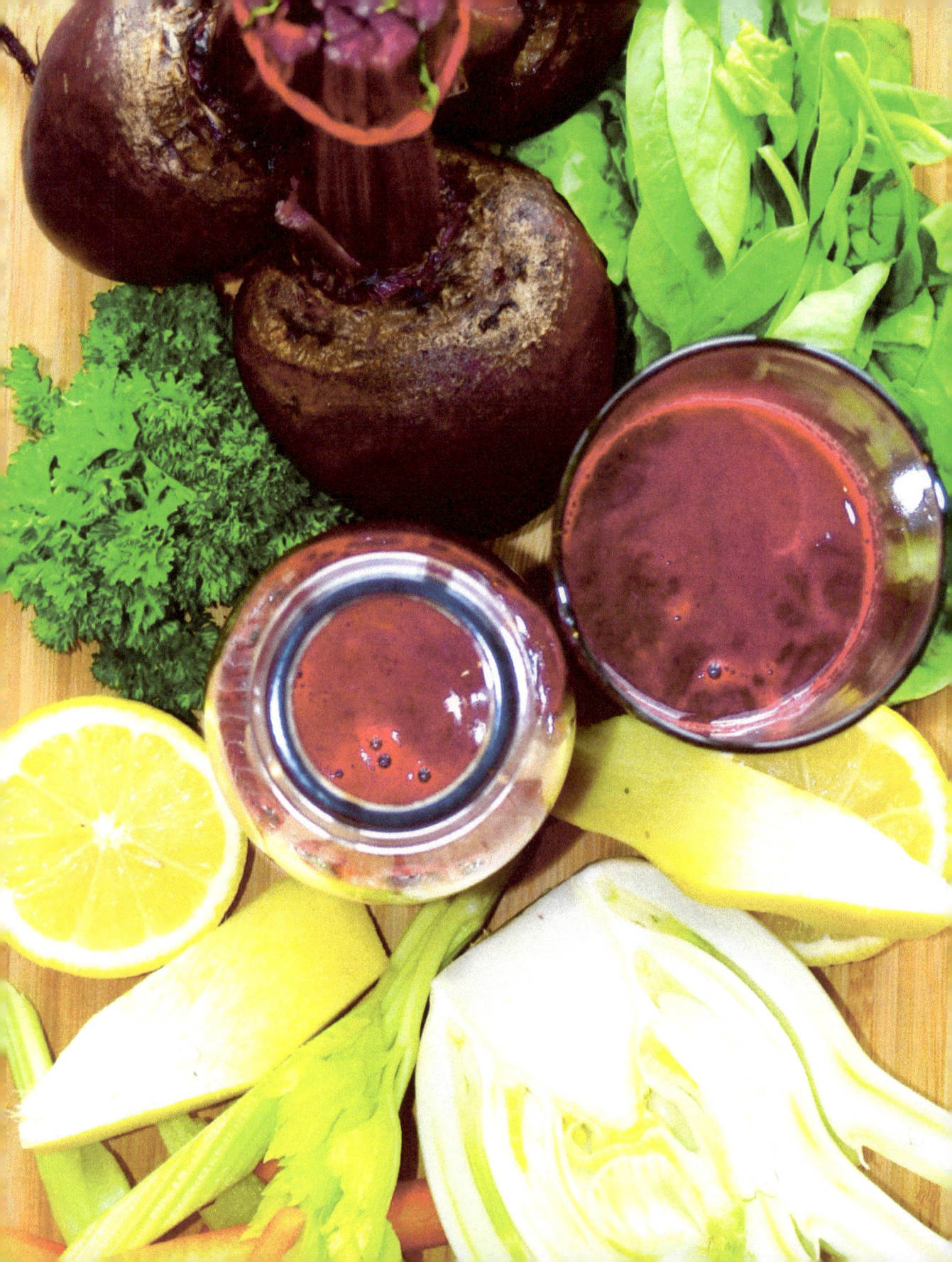

VEGGIE VIT HIT

SERVES 2

3 Medium carrots

1 Rib of celery

½ Fennel bulb

Handful of spinach

Handful of parsley

1 Thumb-size piece of ginger

¼ Lemon

1 Medium Beetroot with stems

Wash & chop celery, fennel, spinach, parsley & lemon into small pieces to fit the shoot of your juicer.

Peel & chop carrots and ginger.

Finally, put on a pair of disposable gloves, then peel & chop the beetroot and stems.

Juice all ingredients through the slow juicer with the sieve in place.

Stir and enjoy.

Beetroot contains a unique group of antioxidants known as betacyanins, it has a liver cleansing action and also promotes good circulation.

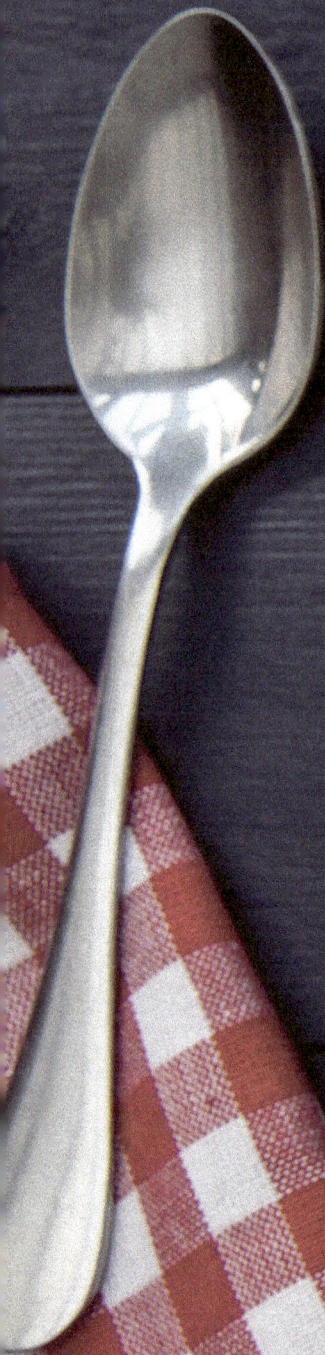

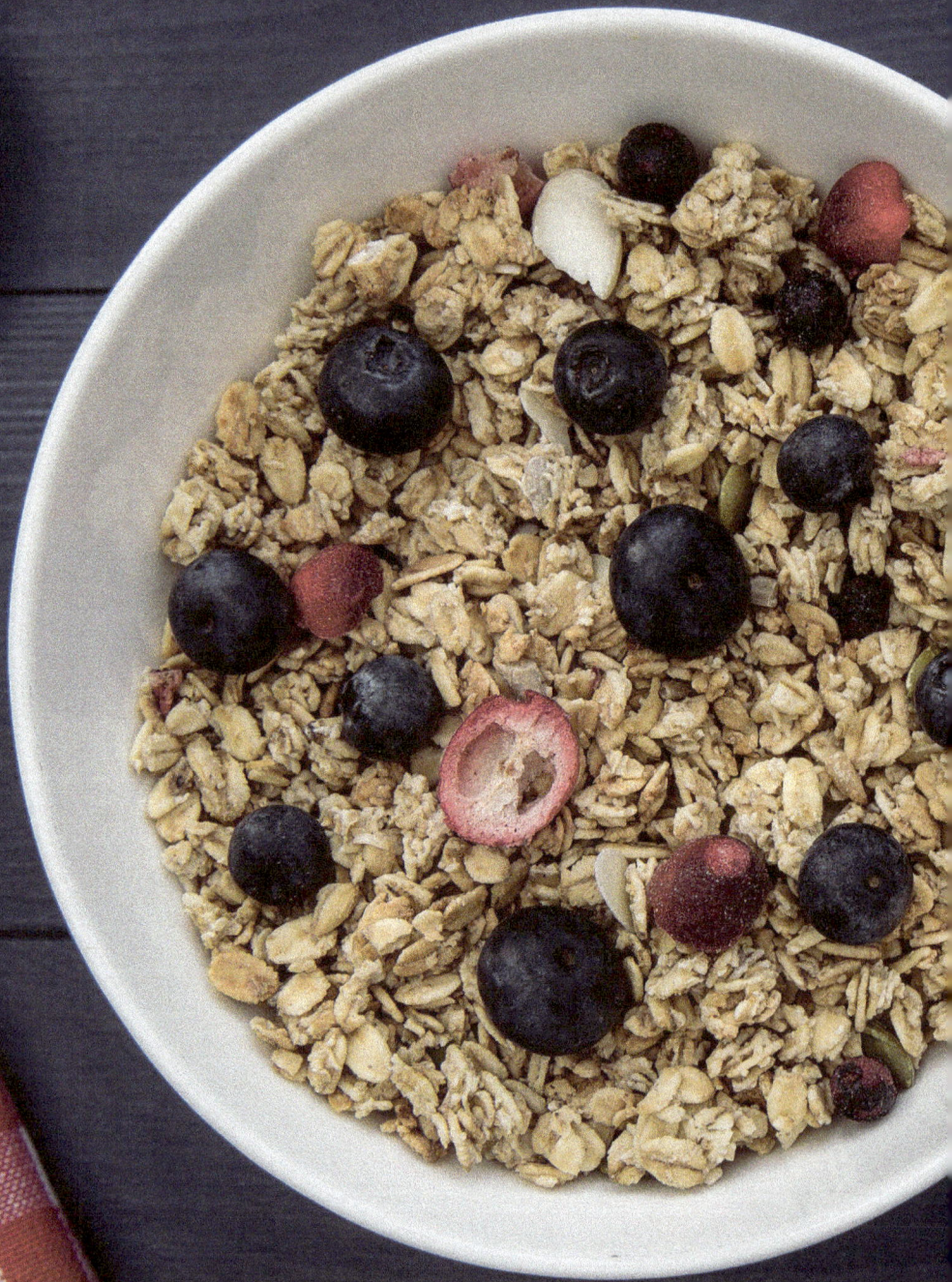

BREAK
THE
FAST

Ideally, we should try to fit our meals in to an
8–10 hour window of the day, for example 8 am –
6 pm, thus allowing a daily 14-hour fast, giving our
gastrointestinal system the time it needs, to fully
digest, absorb and utilise the nutrients in our food.
Hence the term – Break the Fast.

CHILLED OAT & BLUEBERRY "ANGEL DELIGHT"

SERVES 2 – 3

150 grams jumbo organic oats

500 mls boiling water

1 ripe banana

2 tbsp Raw organic local honey

½ tsp cinnamon

200 mls oat milk

100 mls oat crème fraiche

100 grams frozen blueberries

1 tbsp chia seeds

Make a simple porridge with the oats and boiling water in a saucepan, simmer for 5 minutes, take off the heat, transfer into a bowl and chill in the fridge for at least an hour.

Next, put the cold porridge and all of the other ingredients (except chia seeds) into a food processor, and blend until fairly smooth. Serve and garnish with a little extra oat crème fraiche and sprinkle with chia seeds.

Oats are a great source of the water soluble fibre Beta-Glucan which helps maintain healthy cholesterol levels. Oats are also a great food to support your nervous system.

BEANS ON TOAST

SERVES 4-6

1 tbsp extra virgin organic olive oil

1 large onion

1 large sweet potato

500 grams organic tomato passata

70 grams tomato puree

2 tbsp Apple cider vinegar (with the mother culture)

230 grams drained & rinsed cooked cannellini beans (from tin)

230 grams drained & rinsed cooked black beans (from tin)

Ground Himalayan pink salt

1 ripe avocado

Rye bread

Start by preheating your oven to 200 °C. Peel and finely chop the onion, peel and grate the sweet potato.

Place a large non-stick frying pan on a high heat, add the olive oil and the onion, fry for 5 minutes, stirring regularly to prevent burning, add the grated sweet potato and a splash of water, this is called steam frying, the water will quickly evaporate, you may need to add a few more splashes of water whilst you cook and stir the mixture for a further 5 minutes.

Now add the puree, passata & ACV, season to taste with pink salt, lower the heat to medium and stir and cook for another 10 minutes. You can now add the beans, continue to stir the ingredients until evenly distributed. Transfer the beans into a deep baking tray or oven proof dish, place in the oven and bake for 20 minutes.

Remove stone from avocado and scoop flesh into a bowl, add a pinch of salt and mash with a fork until almost pureed.

Toast your rye bread and spread with avocado, serve with your homemade baked beans.

This is a very versatile dish, which can be made in advance and keeps well in the fridge for up to 4 days.

Sweet Potatoes are a great source of potassium which helps regulate heart rate, they can also maintain steady blood sugar levels due to their slow release carbohydrates.

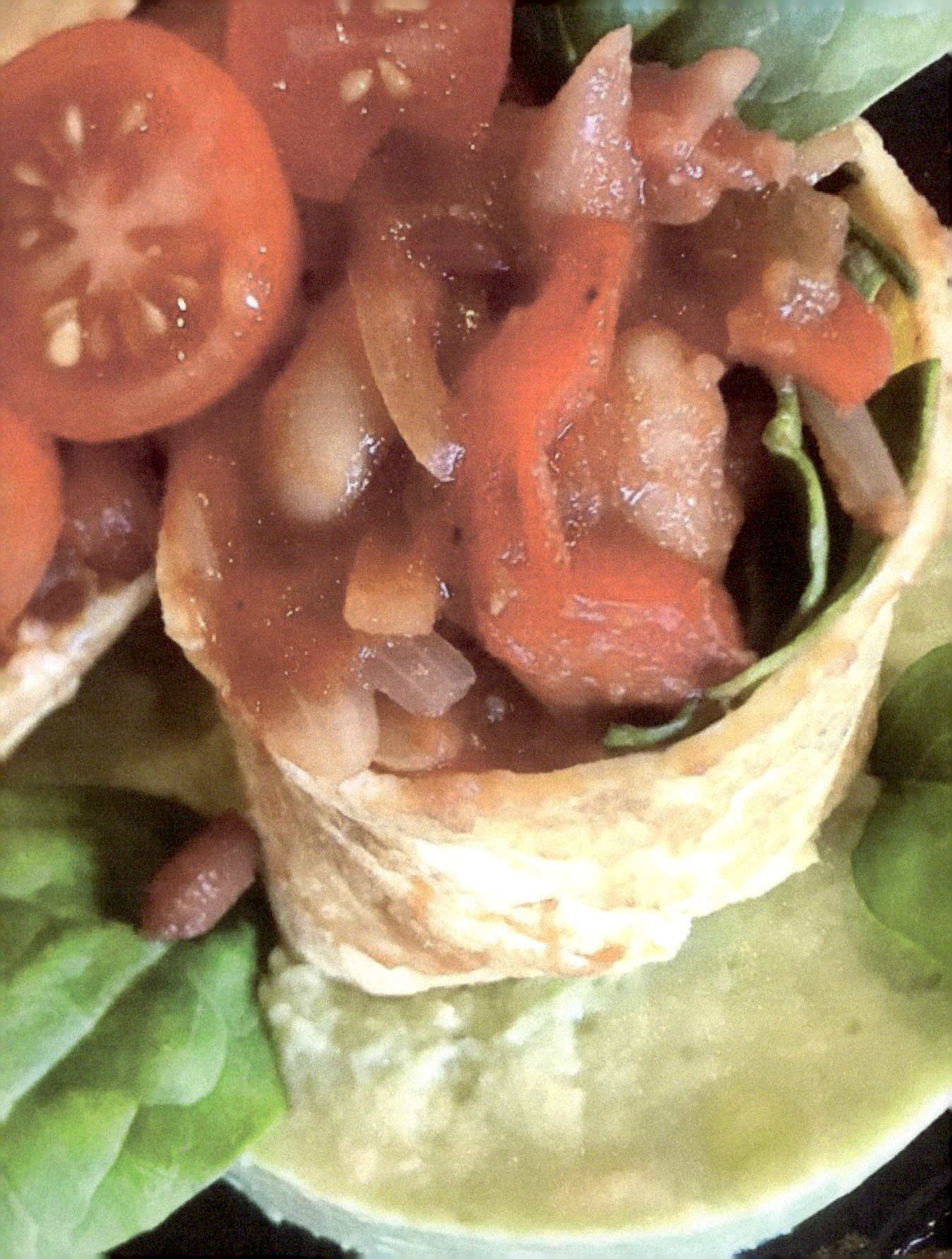

BEAN BURRITO

SERVES 1

2 organic large eggs

1 handful of baby spinach

1 large avocado

1 cup of Mexican mixed beans
(SEE PAGE 77)

Ground Himalayan pink salt

1 tsp extra virgin organic olive oil

Remove stone & skin from avocado, and mash with a pinch of pink salt.

Gently heat the Mexican beans in a small saucepan.

whip together the 2 eggs with a pinch of pink salt. Heat a large non-stick pan, add olive oil to the pan, use a bit of scrunched kitchen paper to smear the oil all over the pan, pour in the eggs, tilting the pan in all directions to make a thin omelette, take off the heat and allow to set and cool slightly.

Flip the omelette onto a large chopping board and turn back over so the more yellow side is facing you. Fill the omelette with the baby spinach and warm beans, and very gently pull in the sides and roll into your burrito shape. I chose to cut mine for the purposes of the picture, however no need to do that.

Spoon your mashed avocado onto a serving plate and place your burrito on top and you're done.

Pulses/beans are a fantastic source of protein and fibre, Including them in your diet is a great way to maintain digestive health and regulate blood sugar levels.

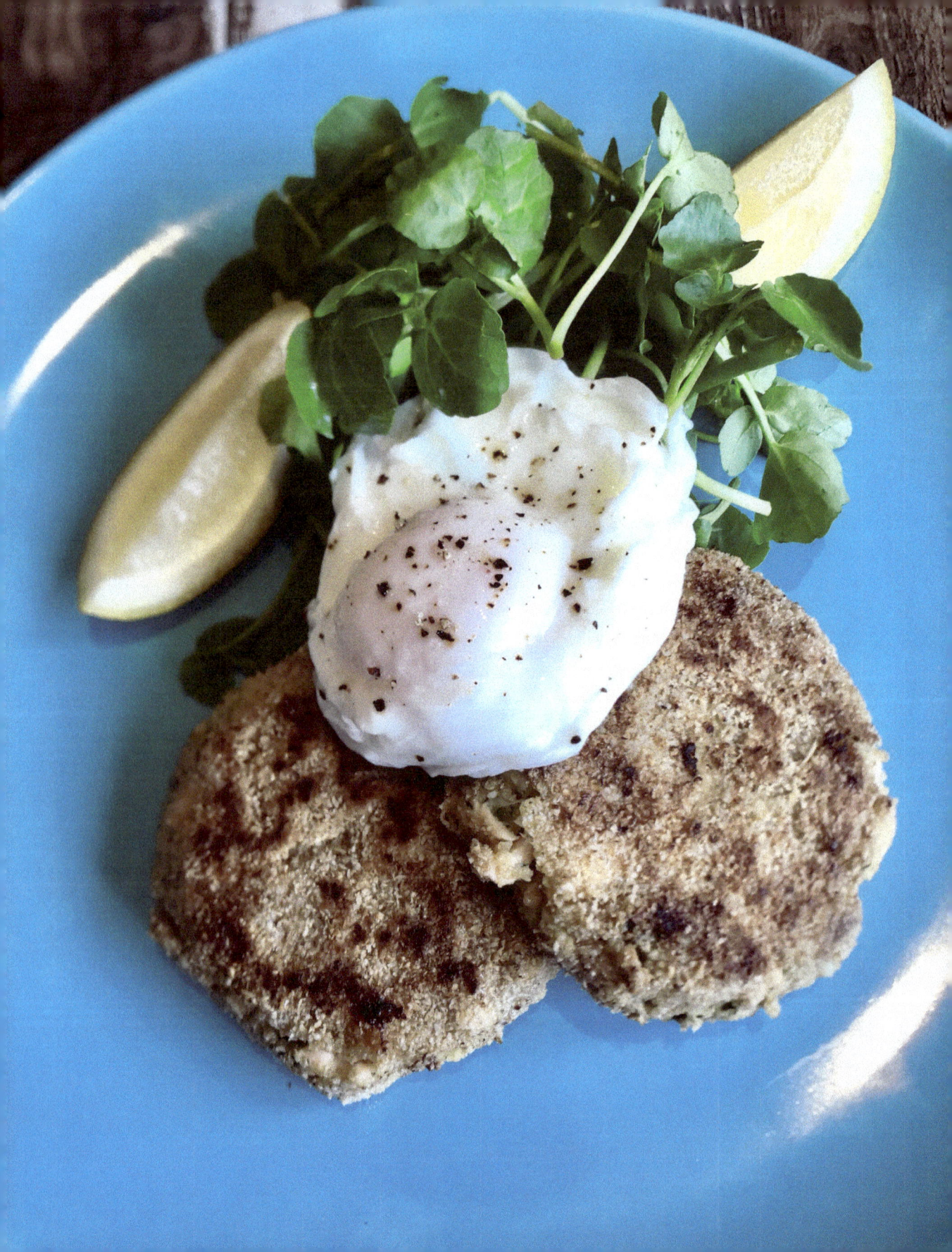

SALMON & DILL FRITTERS WITH POACHED EGG

Serves 4+ (Freezable)

500 grams fresh boneless salmon (preferably belly meat)

250 grams cauliflower florets

175 grams sliced and washed leeks

25 grams chopped dill

zest from 1 unwaxed lemon

2 eggs beaten

oatbran for coating

eggs for poaching

ground Himalayan salt

freshly ground black pepper

watercress

Lemon wedges

1 tbsp extra virgin organic olive oil

Preheat oven to 180 °C, place salmon in an ovenproof dish and season with salt & pepper. Bake salmon for 20 minutes or until just cooked through, remove from oven and leave to cool. Meanwhile boil the cauliflower and leeks together in a saucepan until very tender (mashable). Takes 12 minutes approx. Once cooked, drain through a colander and allow to steam off for 5 minutes, return the cauli and leeks to the pan and mash with a potato masher until you reach a 'mashed potato' consistency, leave to cool. Once the salmon and cauli mash are cool, flake the salmon into a large mixing bowl (leaving in quite large flakes)

add cauli mash, dill, lemon zest and season well with your salt and pepper. Lightly mix all ingredients together and shape into fishcakes (the mix will feel wet at this stage, however the natural fat from the salmon will firm up the fritters when refrigerated). After your fritters are well chilled, you need to coat them. Gently dip the fritters in the beaten egg and then into the oatbran and place back in the fridge. That's all your prep done! Now in the morning preheat a non-stick frying pan, add olive oil, and fry your fritters for 5 minutes each side on a med-high heat. While these are cooking, get your eggs on, poach your eggs in boiling water from the kettle (tip: create a vortex in the water with a whisk and gently crack your egg in which will keep a nice shape to your egg). Serve up with crunchy peppery watercress and garnish with lemon wedges.

Salmon is an oily fish rich in, anti-inflammatory, heart healthy omega-3 essential fatty acids, which supports your cardiovascular system and your nervous system.

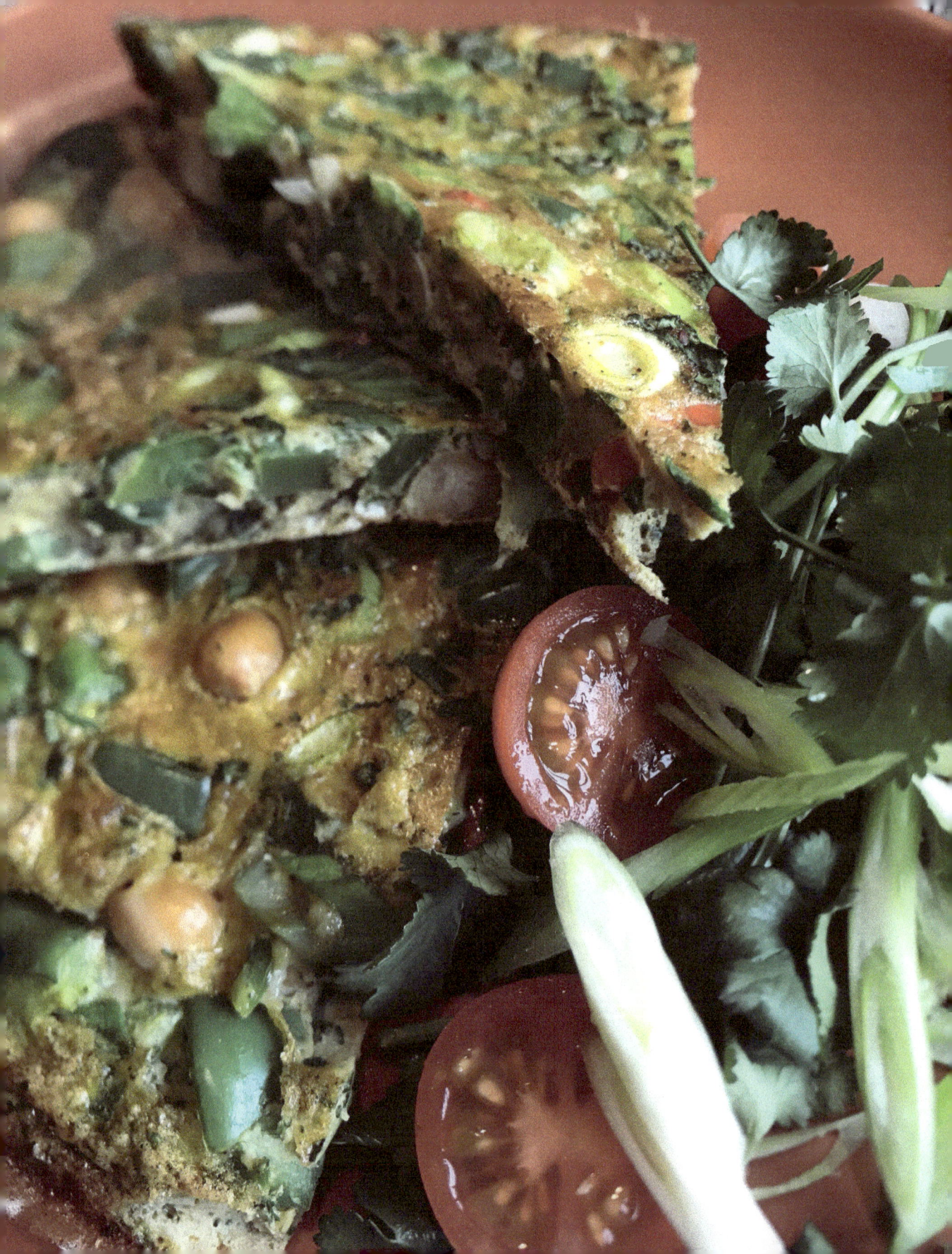

NEW DELHI FRITATTA

SERVES 4

6 Organic large eggs

4 spring onions

25 grams fresh coriander

1 green pepper

130 grams cooked chickpeas (from a can, rinsed)

2 tsp madras curry powder

2 cloves Garlic

½ tsp ginger puree

1 green chilli

1 red chilli

Ground Himalayan pink salt

1 tbsp extra virgin organic olive oil

10 cherry tomatoes

Wash and finely chop spring onion, green pepper, coriander (including stalks), red and green chillies (seeds removed). Mince the garlic and blend with the ginger puree.

Crack your eggs into a large mixing bowl, season well with Himalayan salt, add the curry powder and whisk thoroughly, add all the other ingredients that you have prepared along with the chickpeas and mix well.

Preheat your grill on full power, and place a large non-stick pan on the cooker on a high heat. When the pan is hot add the oil, carefully pour in your egg mixture, ensuring everything is evenly distributed in the pan, leave to cook for 1 minute and then place on the bottom shelf of your grill for a further 5 minutes, or until the frittata is fully cooked and set.

Once cooked, let stand for 1 minute and flip out onto a large chopping board, cut into 8 wedges and serve with sliced cherry tomatoes.

Eggs are an excellent source of quality protein, they also contain vitamin D, necessary for healthy bones and teeth.

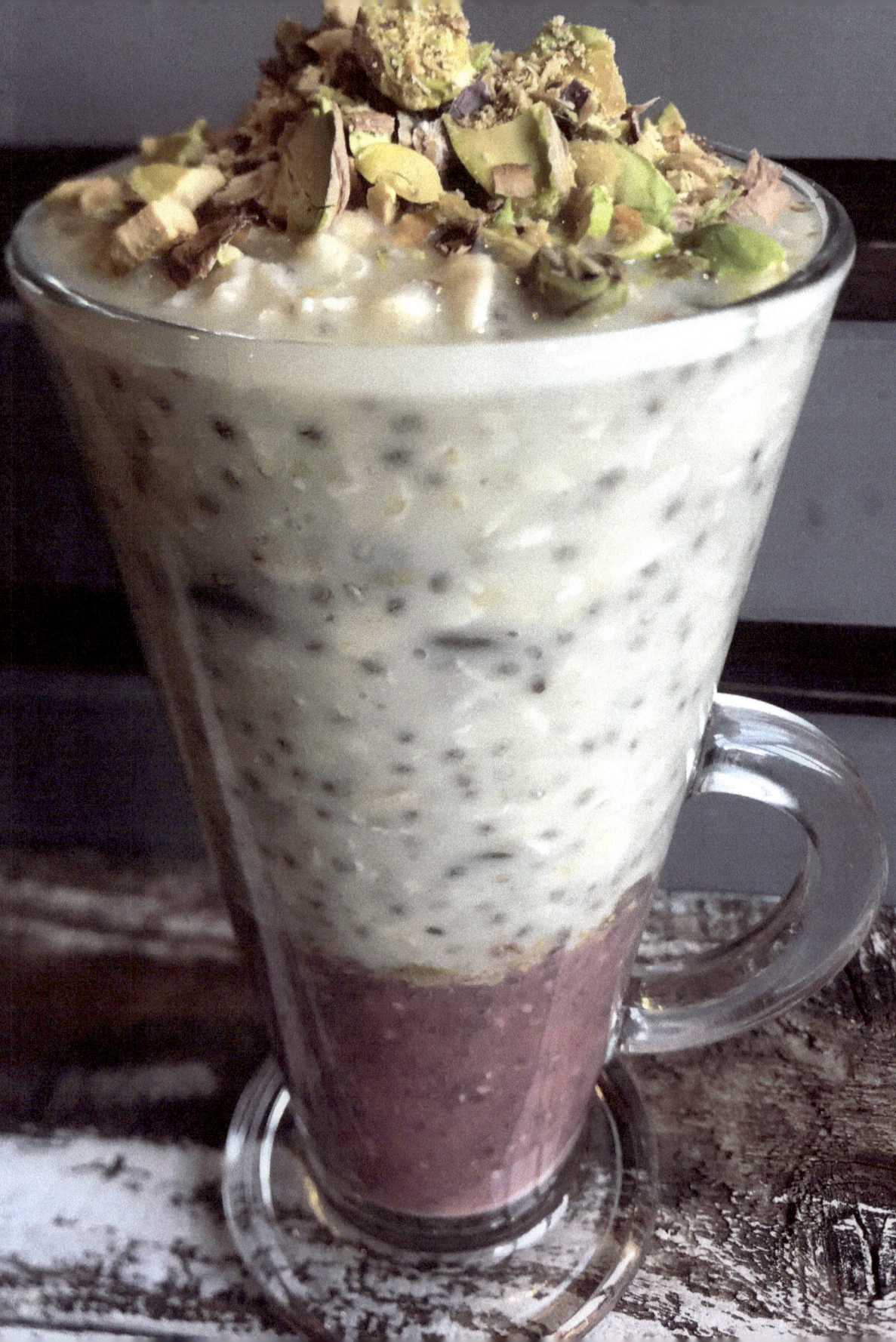

PINEAPPLE, PISTACHIO & PUMPKIN SEED BIRCHER MUESLI WITH STRAWBERRY SURPRISE

SERVES 2

¼ of a peeled ripe pineapple roughly chopped (including core)

1 granny smith apple

1 ripe banana

300 mls oat milk

1 cup of jumbo organic oats

¼ cup of chia seeds + 1 tbsp chia seeds

¼ cup pumpkin seeds

20 grams crushed pistachio nuts

6 large strawberries

Wash, core and chop apple, place in your nutri-bullet with banana, pineapple & oat milk, blend for 1 minute.

Put your oats, pumpkin seeds & ¼ cup chia seeds into a mixing bowl, and pour over your Pineapple, apple and banana milk, stir well and place in fridge for at least 1 hour.

Meanwhile, blitz your strawberries in the nutri-bullet for 1 minute, then add the 1 tbsp chia seeds and mix well, pour your strawberry surprise into your serving glasses and place in fridge alongside your bircher muesli.

After 1 hour, both mixtures will have firmed up somewhat. Sprinkle in some crushed pistachios on top of the strawberry layer and then top up with the bircher muesli. Finally garnish with the remaining pistachios.

This recipe can be made in advance and keeps well in the fridge for 2-3 days.

Chia seeds are high in omega-3, protein, fibre, calcium and magnesium. They promote normal bowel regularity and are naturally detoxifying.

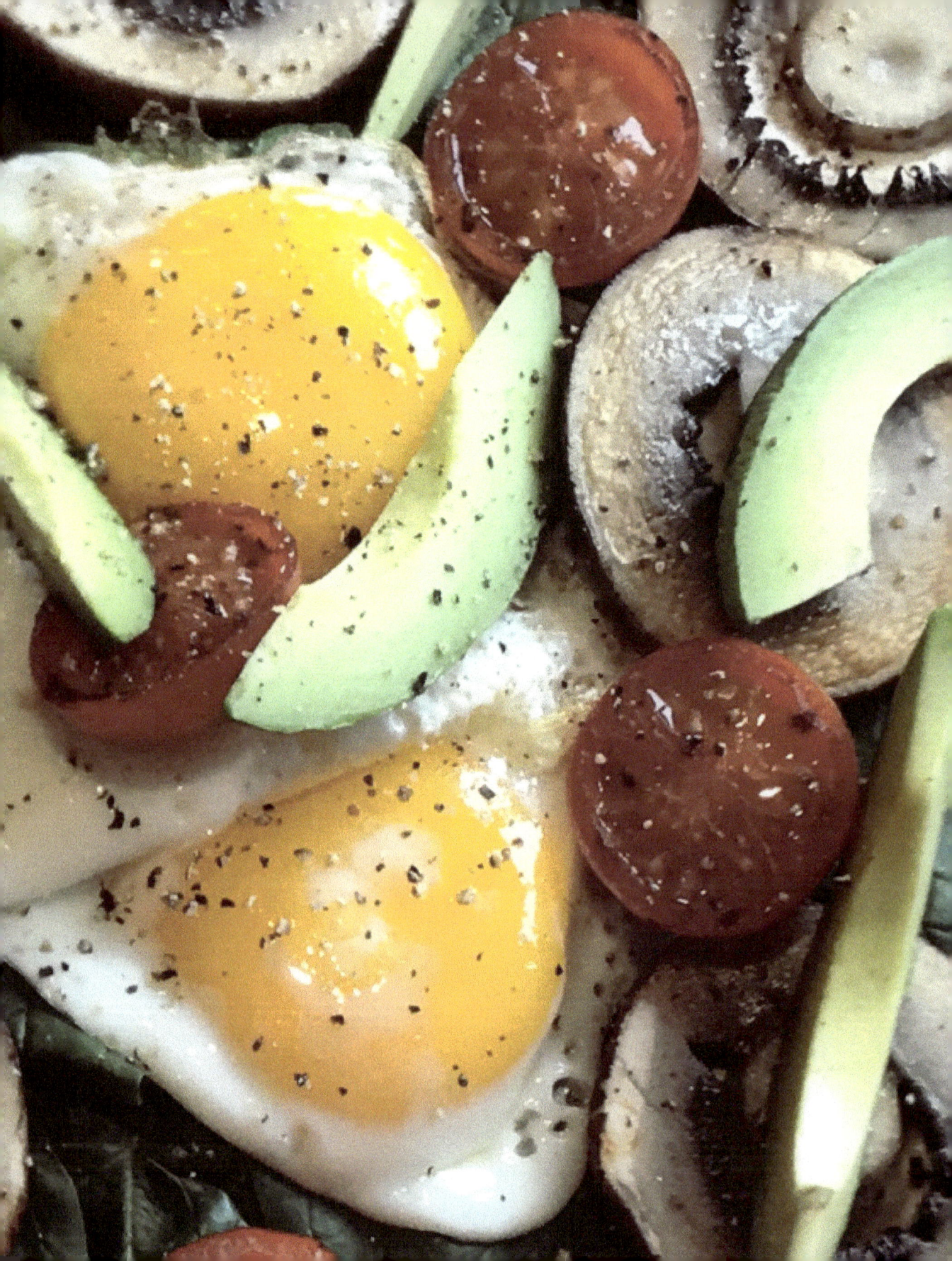

SERVES 1

1 small handful of washed baby spinach

4 vine cherry tomatoes

4 large chestnut mushrooms

½ ripe avocado

2 organic eggs

1 slice rye bread

1 tbsp extra virgin organic olive oil

ground Himalayan pink salt

freshly ground black pepper

Wash and cut the tomatoes in half, use a pastry brush to remove any dirt from mushrooms and cut in half, place on a baking tray, season with salt & pepper and put under a hot grill for 5 minutes approx.

Meanwhile arrange the spinach on your serving plate and get a non-stick frying pan on a high heat, add 1 tbsp olive oil, crack in the eggs and cook to your liking.

Prepare the avocado by removing stone & skin, and thinly slice.

Put your rye bread in the toaster and arrange everything else on your serving plate.

Finally place the finished plate under the hot grill for 30 seconds to ensure everything is warm and serve with your rye toast.

Avocado contains beneficial monounsaturated oils which can help lower blood pressure and lubricate joints.

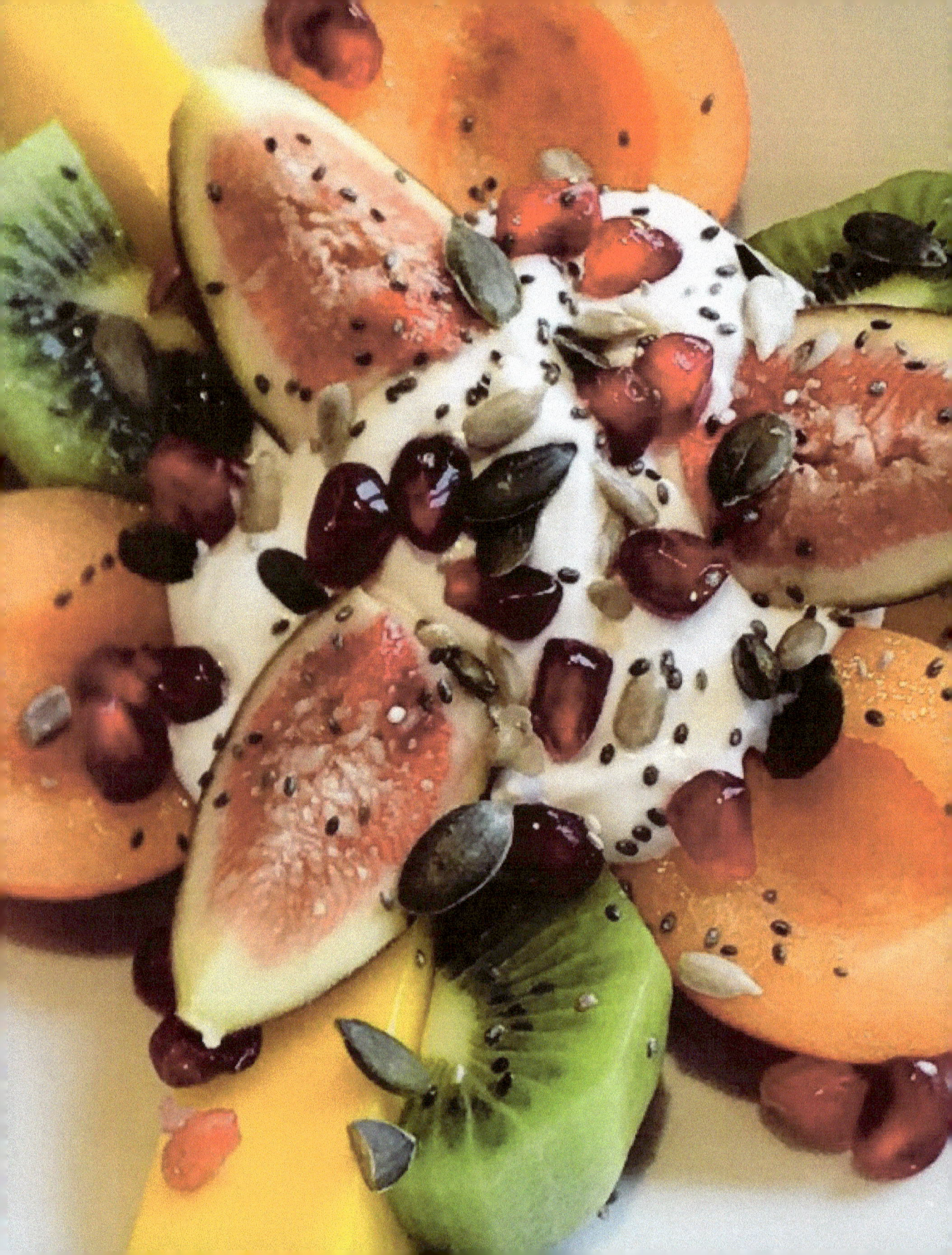

SEASONAL FRUITS WITH COCONUT YOGHURT & SEEDS

2 Fresh figs

2 fresh apricots

1 kiwi

½ ripe mango

pomegranite seeds

pumkin seeds

sunflower seeds

chia seeds

coconut yoghurt

Wash, trim and quarter figs, cut apricots in half and remove stone, peel and slice kiwi, peel and cut mango into wedges.

Arrange your fruits in a serving bowl, add a dollop of coconut yoghurt, sprinkle over your seeds and enjoy.

Mangoes boost the immune system helping reduce the incidence of colds and flu.

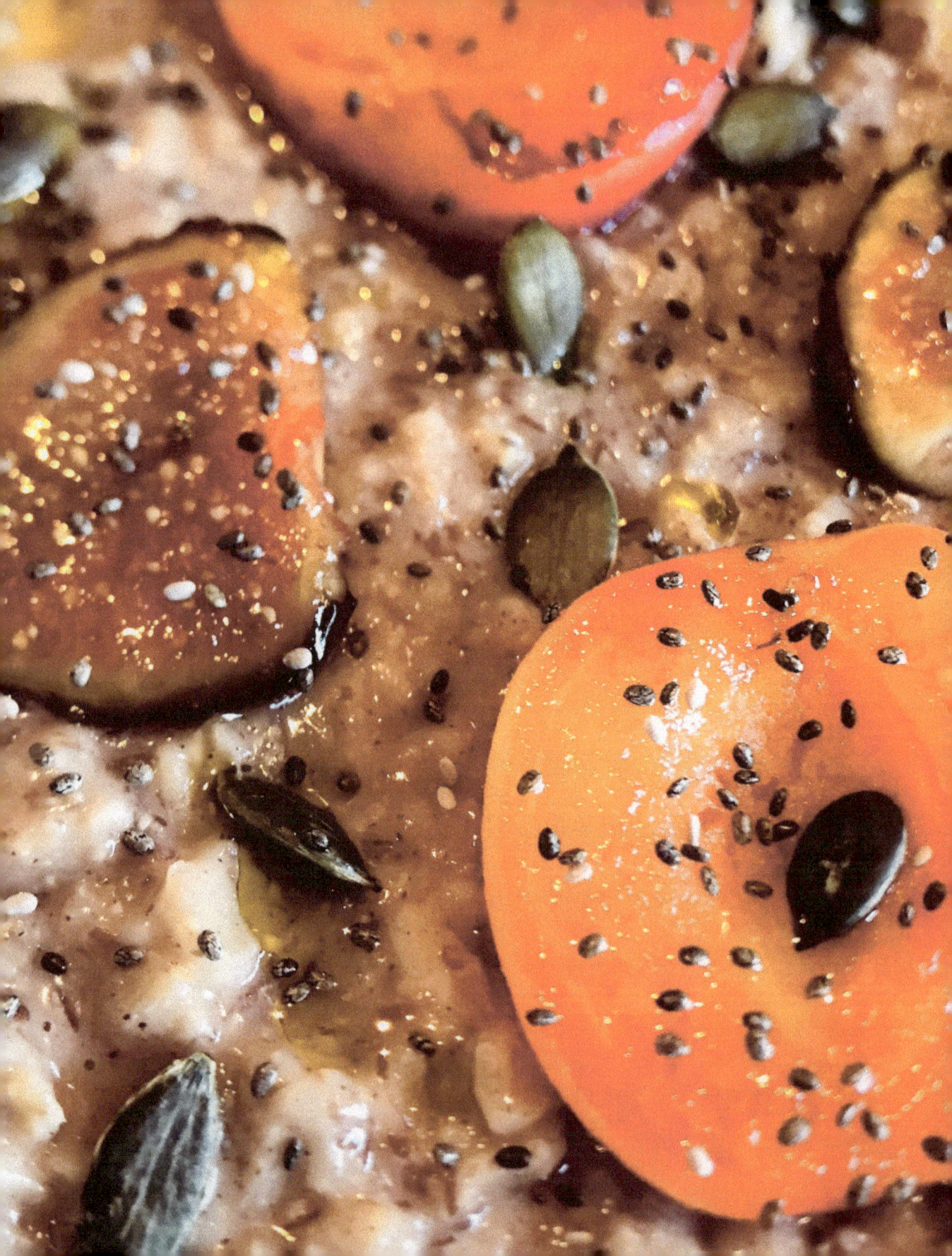

HOT PORRIDGE WITH HONEY-GLAZED APRICOTS & FIGS

SERVES 1

½ cup jumbo organic oats

1 cup of boiling water

½ cup of oatmilk

1 tbsp ground flaxseed

1 tsp flaxseed oil or olive oil

½ tsp ground cinnamon

1 tbsp date syrup

½ tsp coconut oil

1 fresh fig

1 fresh apricot

1 tbsp organic local raw honey

1 tsp pumpkin seeds

¼ tsp chia seeds

Cook your oats with the boiling water in a medium saucepan for 4–5 minutes or until the oats have popped and puffed. Add the ground flaxseed, cinnamon, date syrup & oat milk, mix well and bring back to the boil, then remove from the heat.

Place a non-stick frying pan on a high heat, cut your apricot in half, remove stone, cut your fig in half too, add your coconut oil to the pan followed by the fruits, flesh side down. Fry for 1 minute each side, until lightly coloured, then add the honey and allow to sizzle for 30 seconds, then remove from the heat.

Serve your porridge in a warm bowl. Top with the glazed fruits and sprinkle with pumpkin and chia seeds.

Apricots have high levels of vitamin a which promotes healthy eyes and skin.

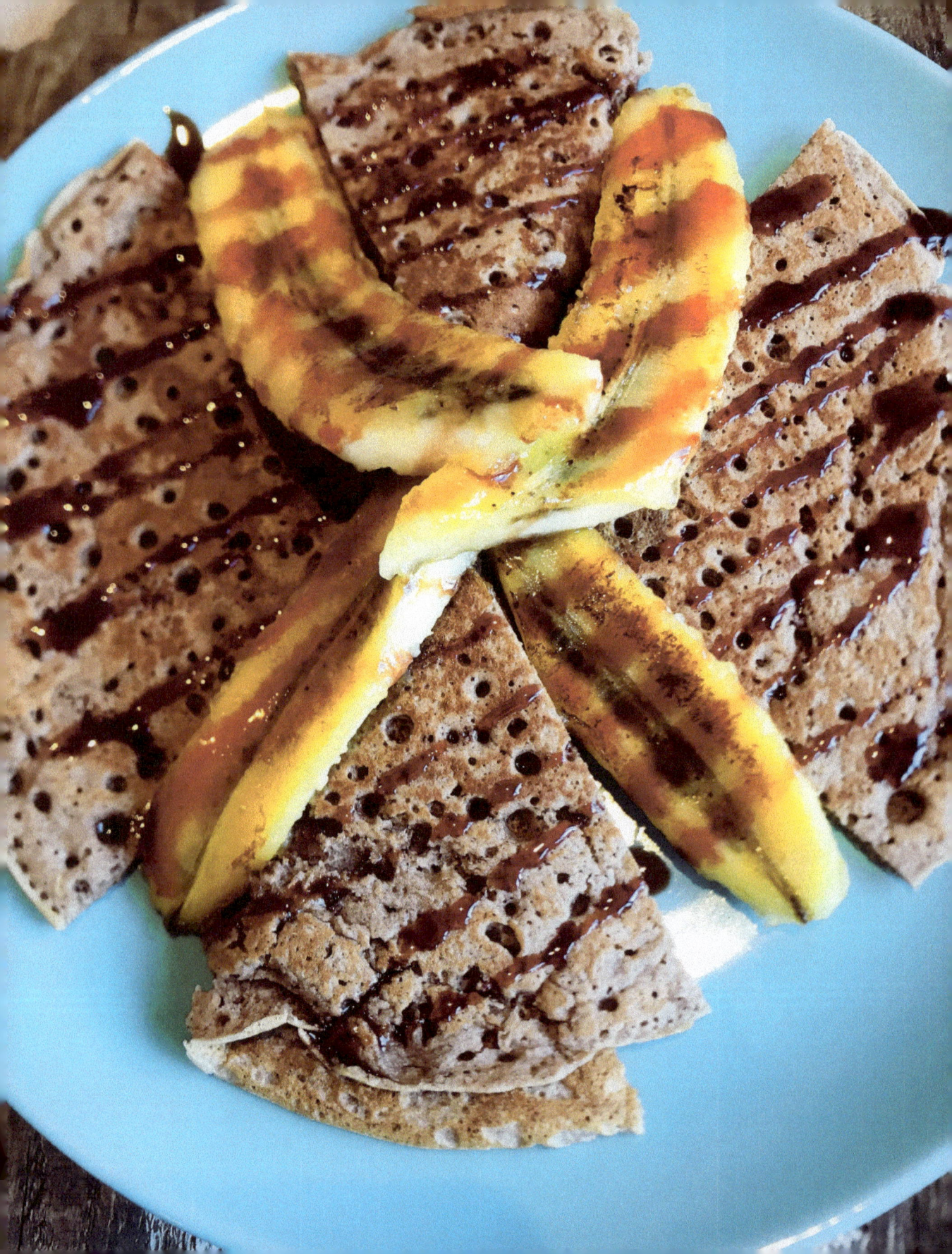

WHOLEMEAL SPELT PANCAKES WITH CARAMELISED BANANA

MAKES 5 LARGE PANCAKES –
1 PANCAKE = 1 PORTION

2 cups organic wholemeal spelt flour

2 cups coconut milk alternative

2 tbsp melted coconut oil & more for cooking

1 organic egg

4 tsp baking powder

pinch of Himalayan pink salt

3 tbsp date syrup + more for drizzling

1 tbsp ground cinnamon

1 large banana per portion

1 tbsp organic local raw honey

Crack the egg into a large mixing bowl and beat well with a whisk. Add the flour, baking powder, coconut milk, cinnamon, salt & date syrup and whisk to a smooth consistency. Now pour in the melted coconut oil and continue to whisk until fully incorporated in the mixture.

Place an 11.5 inch non-stick frying pan on a high heat. Add a little coconut oil, pour in 1 medium sized ladle of the mixture, tilt the pan in all directions until the mixture has covered the complete surface of the pan. Now leave to cook for 1–2 minutes. bubbles will start to appear on top. Shake the pan to release the pancake, you may need to use a fish slice to assist the releasing. Once the pancake is freely sliding, it's time for the flip. You can use a large fish slice to help you flip the pancake or if you're confident, toss and flip the pancake using the pan handle. Repeat this process until all your batter is finished.

Meanwhile, peel and slice the banana into long strips. Give your frying pan a quick wipe and place back on the heat, add a little coconut oil and fry the banana for 1-2 minutes each side. To achieve a little caramelisation, add the honey, allow to sizzle for 20–30 seconds and remove from the heat.

You can reheat the pancake in hot oven if you wish for 1 minute, Serve 1 pancake with the banana and drizzle with more date syrup.

Bananas are very high in Potassium and fibre which support the normal function of the gastrointestinal and cardiovascular systems.

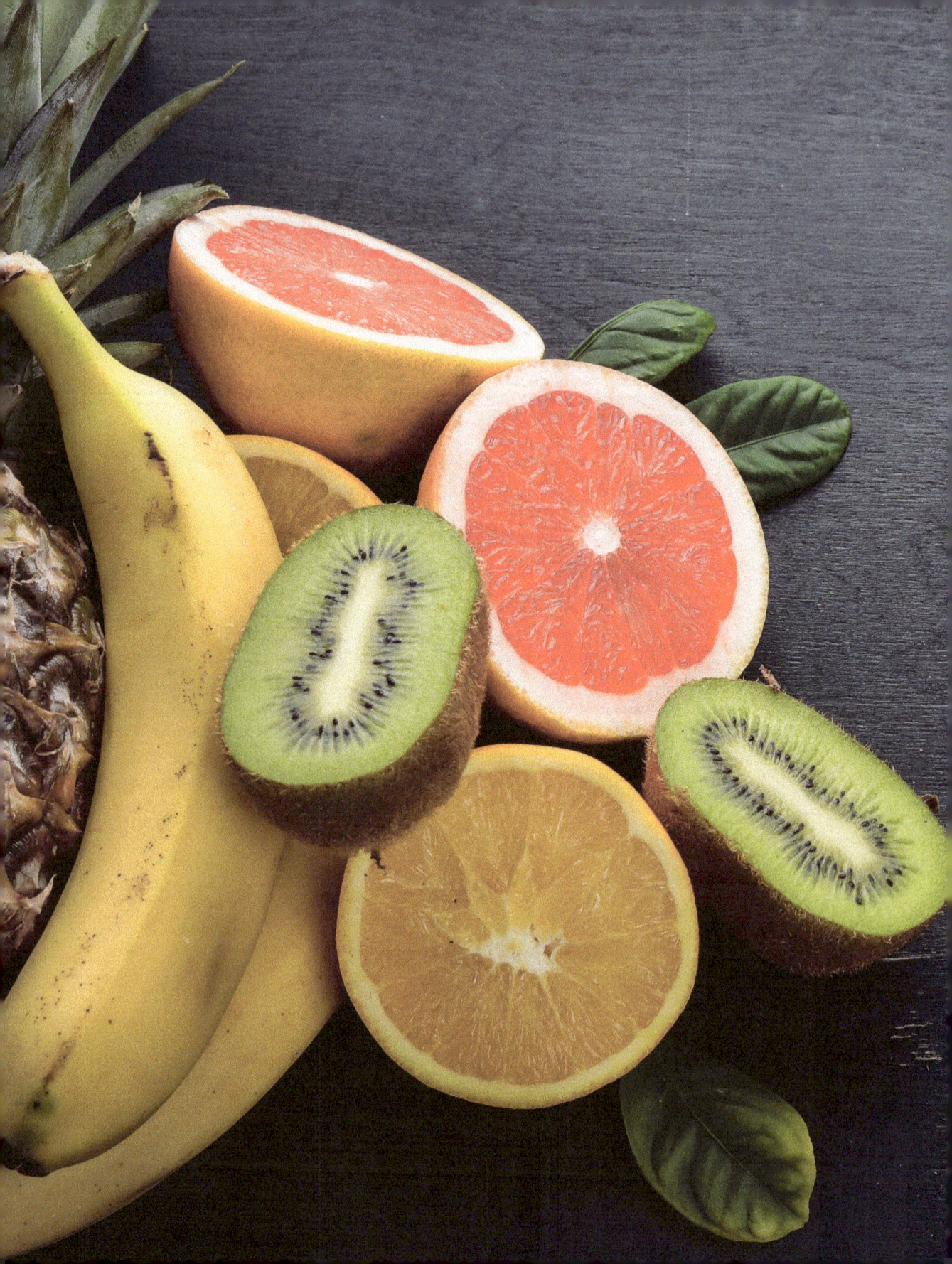

SUPER SMOOTHIES

Smoothies are a great convenient way of loading up on nutrients, especially for people with very busy lifestyles. They can be used as a snack or even a meal replacement on the odd occasion, giving great flexibility when planning your meals. I strongly recommend incorporating a source of protein to any smoothie.

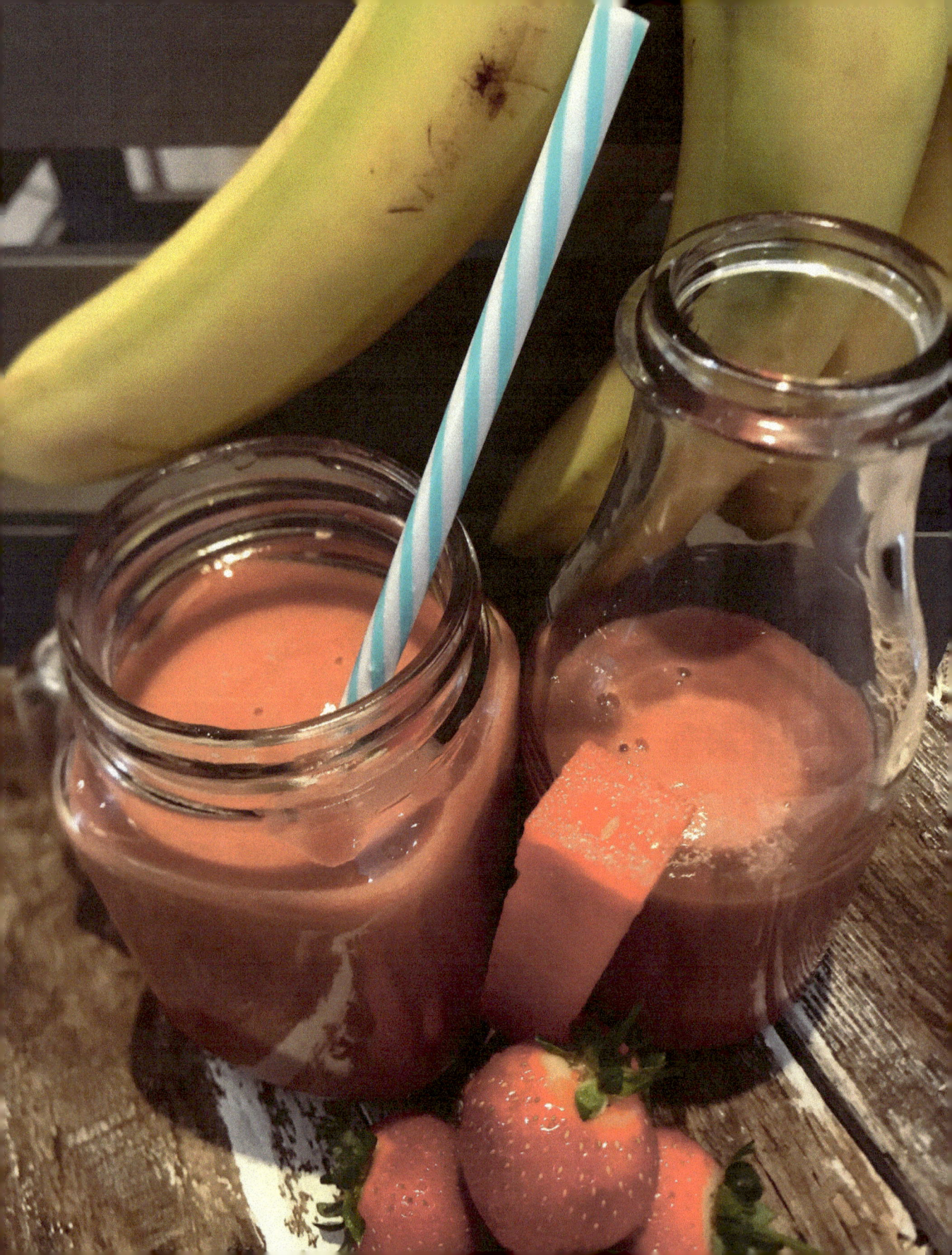

THE RED ONE

SERVES 2

200 grams of watermelon

200 grams of fresh organic strawberries

100 grams of tomato passata

1/3 cup of pea protein powder

coconut water

Place all ingredients in the nutri-bullet and pour in enough coconut water until you reach the fill line.

Blend for 1 minute and serve.

Organic Strawberries are a source of manganese and iodine, which support the normal function of the thyroid.

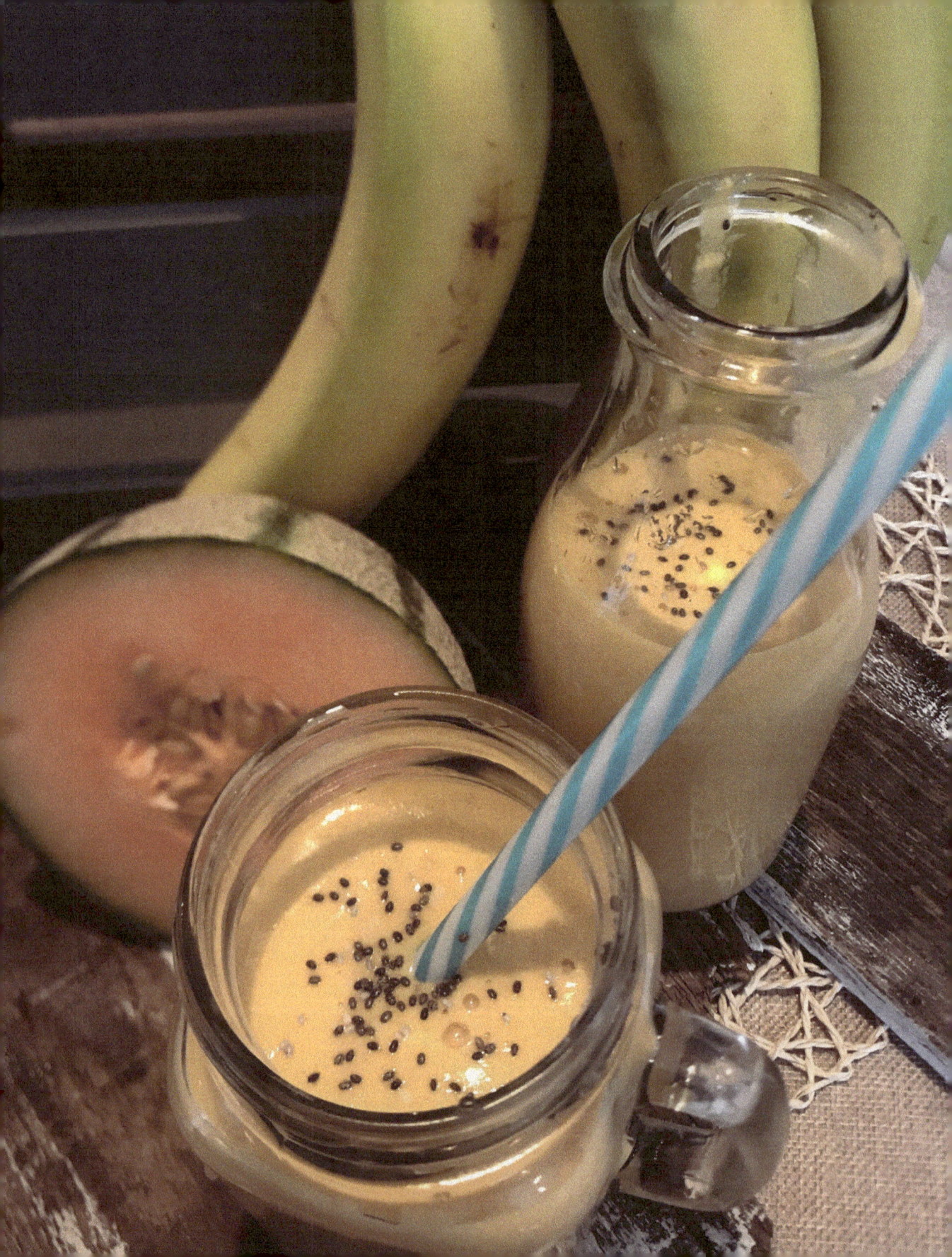

THE ORANGE ONE

SERVES 2

100 grams of cooked carrots

100 grams of frozen mango chunks

100 grams of cantaloupe melon

1 level scoop of pea protein powder

1 thumb-size piece of ginger minced

freshly squeezed orange juice

Place all ingredients in the nutri-bullet, pour in orange juice up to the fill line. Blitz for 1 minute.

Garnish with chia seeds (optional).

Cantaloupe melon is the most nutrient dense melon containing high levels of vitamin A and C which supports your immune system.

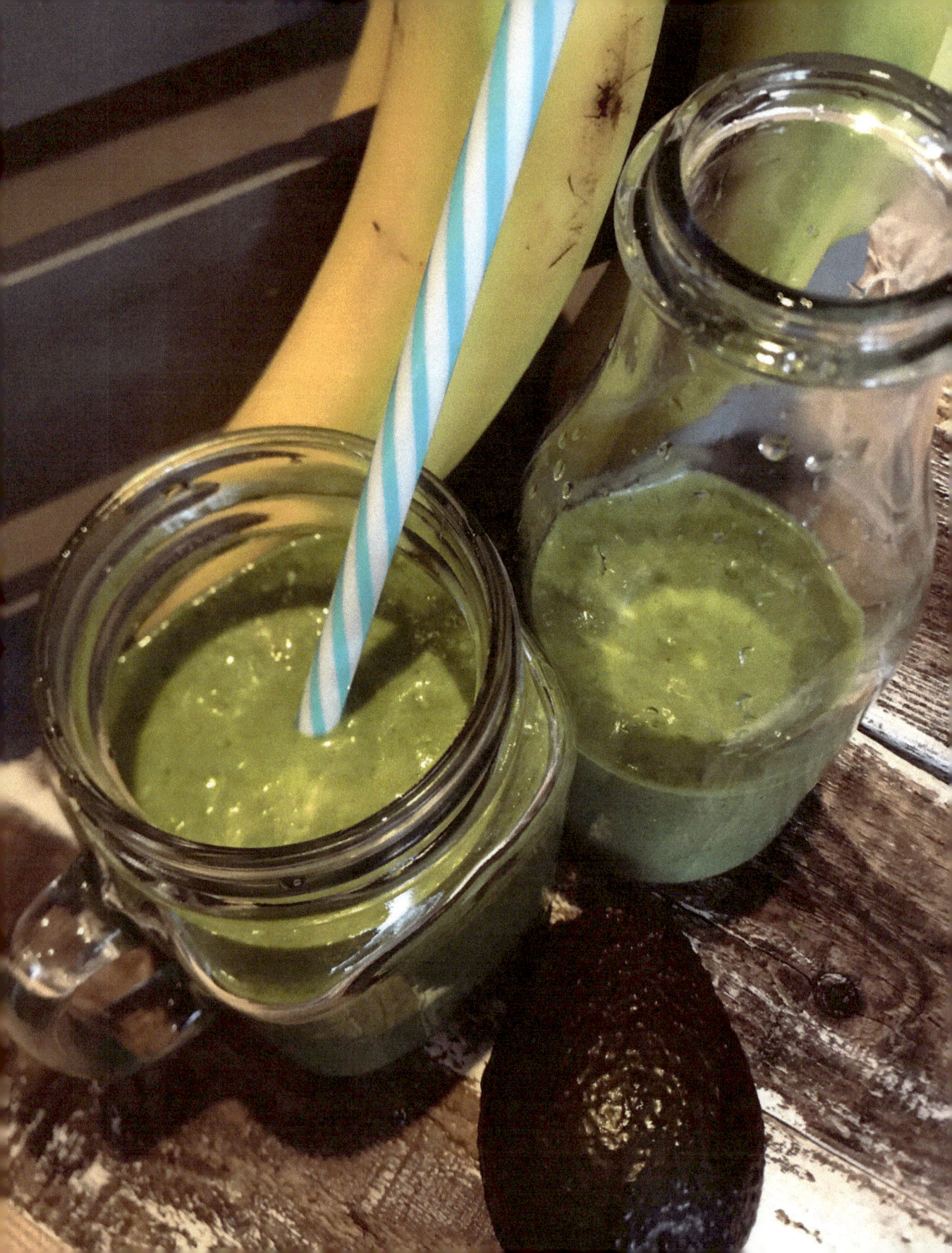

THE GREEN ONE

SERVES 2

1 large handful of frozen kale

1 handful of frozen parsley

1 small avocado

½ banana

1/3 cup of pea protein powder

fresh pressed apple juice

Place all ingredients in the nutri-bullet and pour apple juice up to the fill line.

Blitz for 1 minute and serve.

Kale is jam packed with vitamins and minerals that help fight inflammation, strengthen bones and balance hormones.

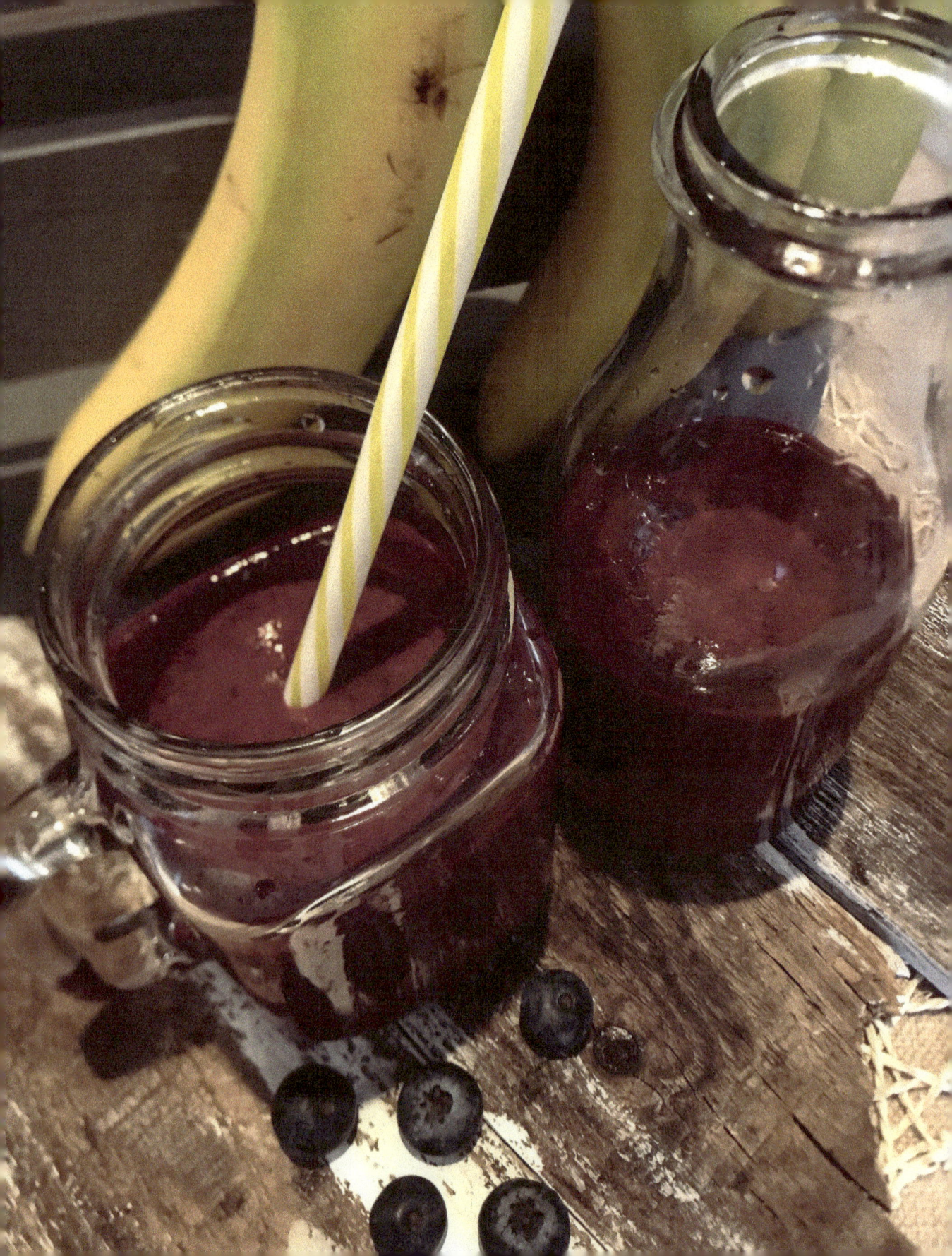

THE PURPLE ONE

SERVES 2

100 grams of steamed beetroot

100 grams of fresh blueberries

100 grams of acai pulp puree (sambazon)

½ banana

1/3 cup of pea protein powder

fresh pressed apple juice

Place all ingredients in the nutri-bullet, pour in apple juice up to the fill line.

Blitz for 1 minute and serve.

Acai berry has the highest antioxidant content of any fruit or vegetable, which helps fight the aging process, reduces inflammation and aids in weight loss.

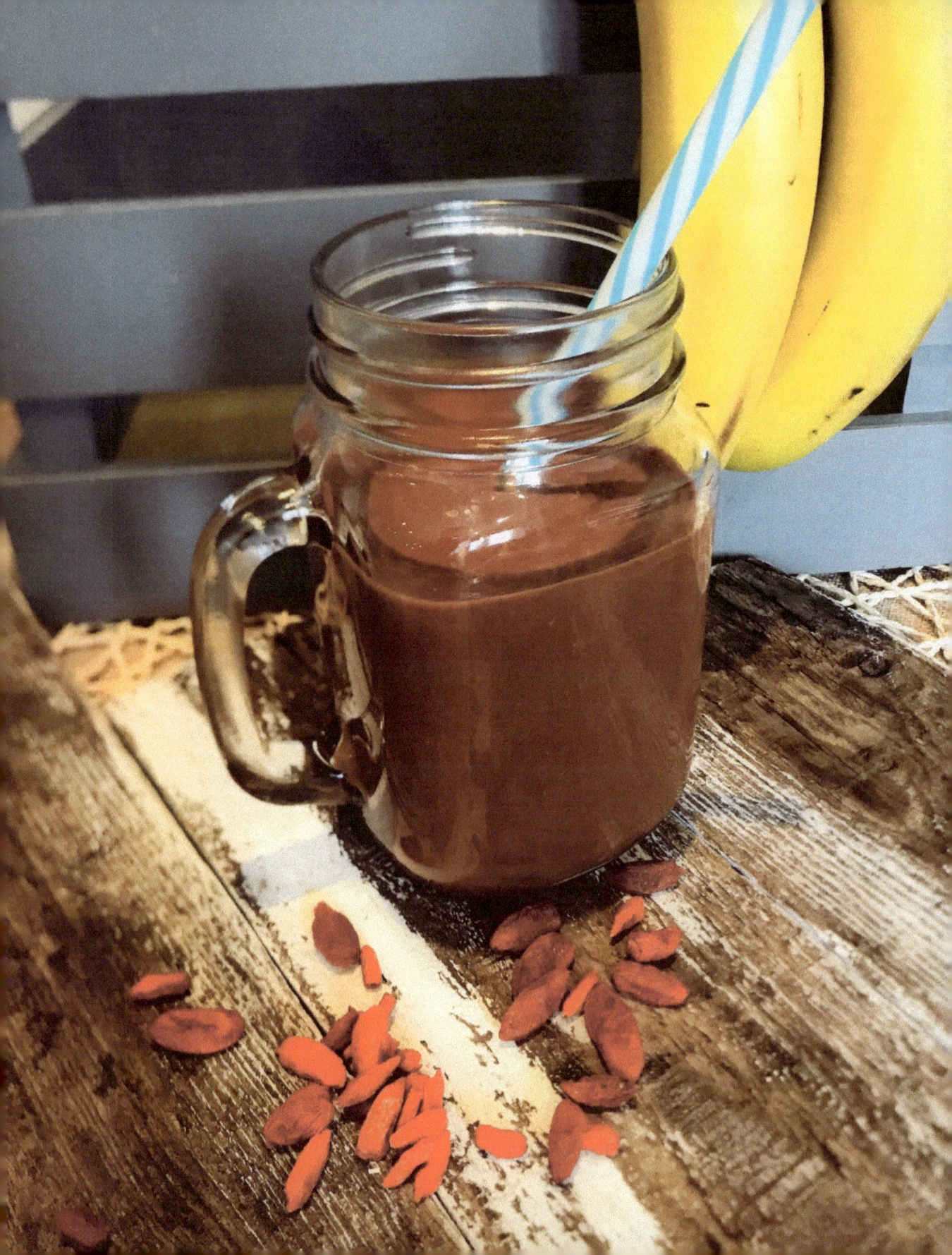

SIMPLE SUPERFOOD SMOOTHIE

SERVES 2

1/3 cup Goji berries

1 heaped tbsp maca powder

2 heaped tbsp cacao powder

1 heaped tbsp Baobab powder

½ tsp cinnamon

oatmilk

coconut water

Place dry ingredients in the nutri-bullet cup and fill to the max line with 50/50 oatmilk & coconut water.

Blitz for 1 minute and serve

Goji berries contain around 10 times the antioxidant capacity of blueberries, helping supply oxygen to your cells, promote peaceful sleep and healthy skin.

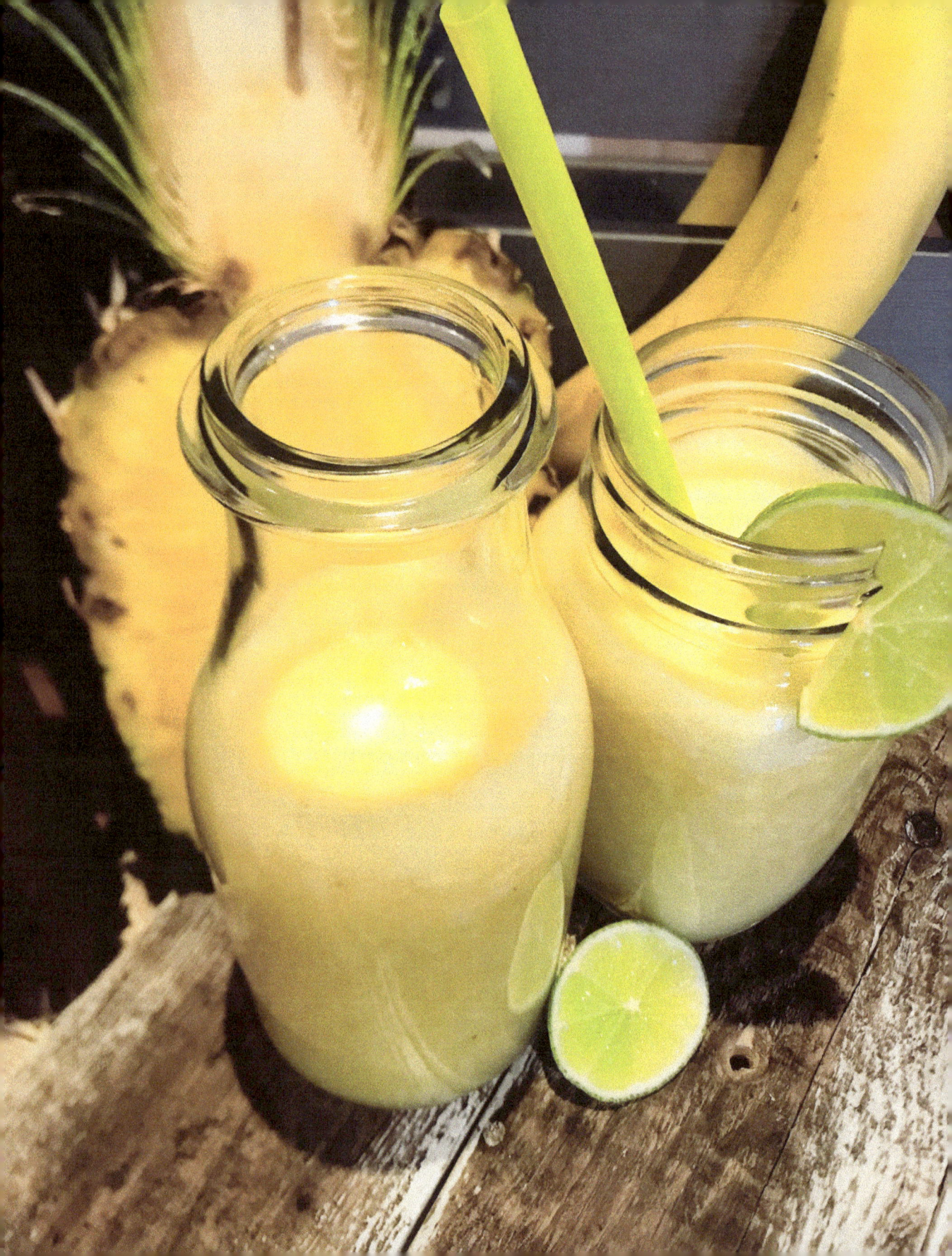

TROPICAL PINEAPPLE BREEZER

SERVES 2

½ Medium pineapple (peeled with core intact)

1 banana

Juice of half of lime

2 frozen lemon & ginger cubes
(SEE PAGE 5)

Coconut water

Peel and roughly chop the pineapple (don't remove core)

Peel and roughly chop banana

Place in the nutri-bullet with lemon and ginger cubes, lime juice and add coconut water to the max line.

Blitz for 1 minute and serve

Coconut water is excellent for Maintaining electrolyte levels & can help reduce fatigue, stress and help maintain muscle relaxation.

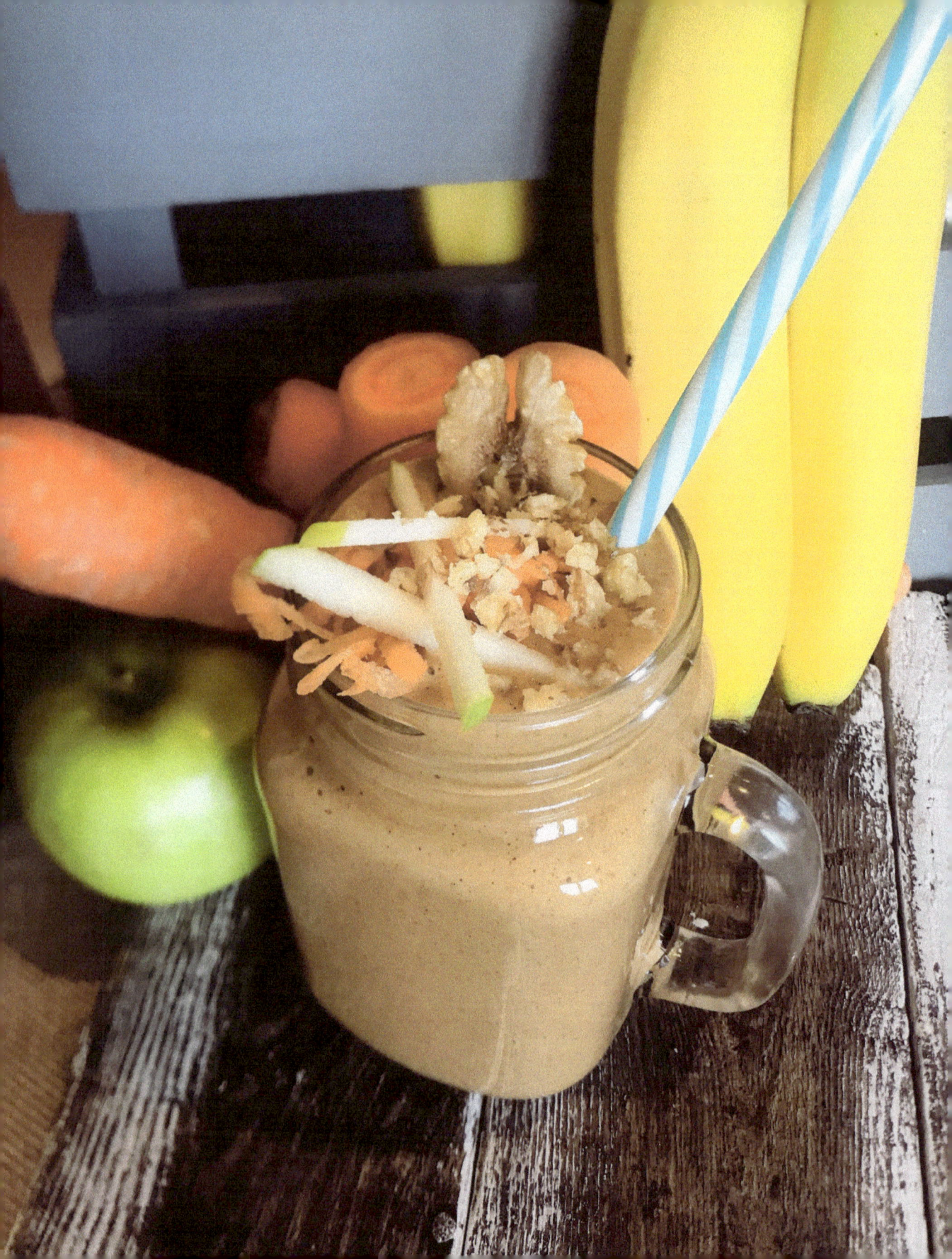

CARROT CAKE SMOOTHIE

SERVES 2

1 medium sized carrot (grated)

2 small bananas

20 walnut halves (soaked in water overnight)

1 tbsp ground flaxseed

2 tbsp organic sugar free apple puree

1 tsp cinnamon

½ tsp ground nutmeg

1 tsp organic vanilla paste

fresh cold pressed carrot juice

Place all ingredients into your nutri-bullet cup and fill to the max line with the carrot juice.

Blitz for 1 minute and serve

Walnuts contain serotonin, they are the perfect brain food.

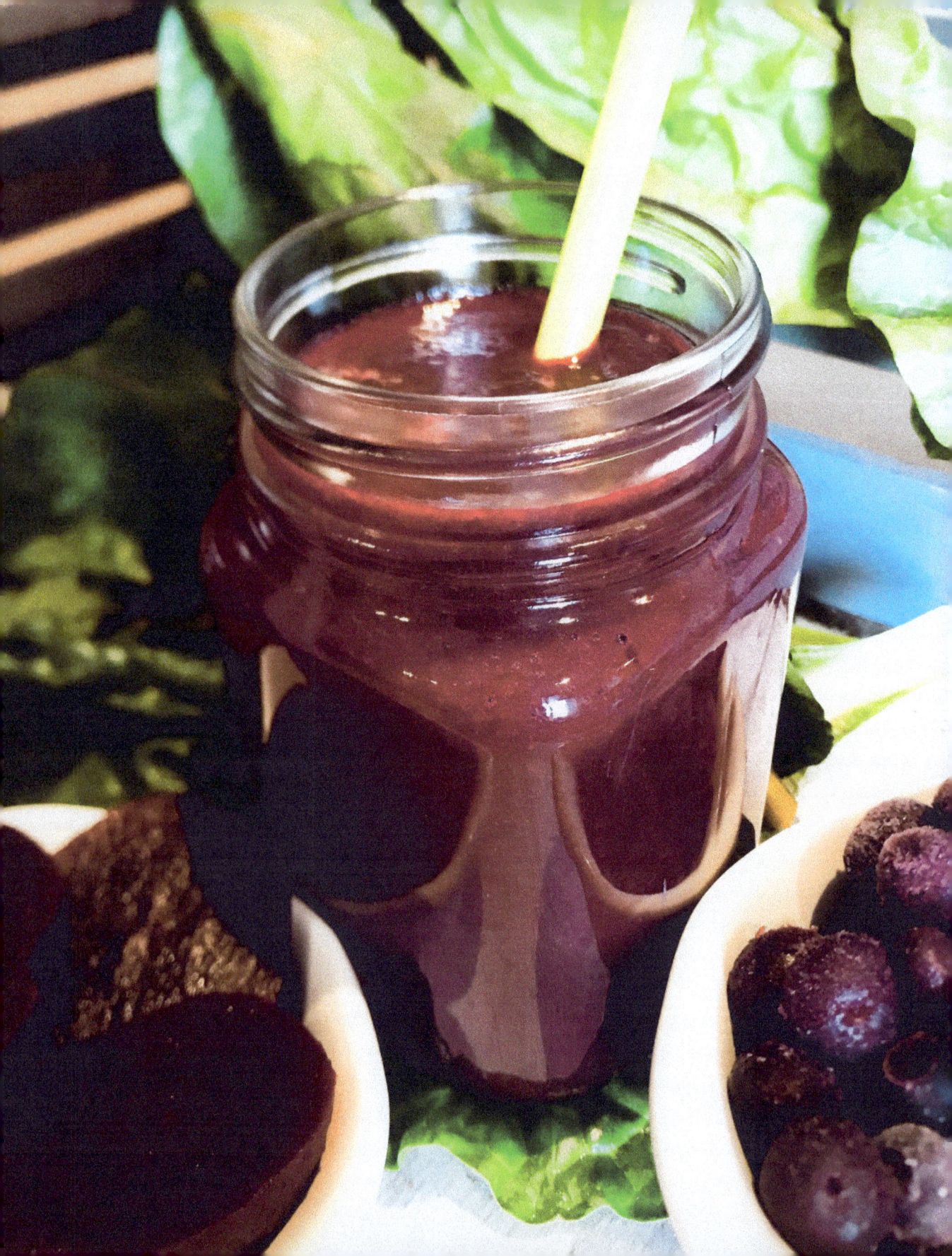

BERRY BEET SMOOTHIE

SERVES 2

170 grams steamed beetroot

50 grams rainbow chard

100 grams frozen blueberries

Cold pressed Beetroot juice

Wash and roughly chop the rainbow chard, place in your nutri-bullet cup along with the beetroot and frozen blueberries.

Fill to the max line with the beetroot juice.

Blitz for 1 minute and serve.

Blueberries contain certain antibacterial antioxidants which promote a healthy gut.

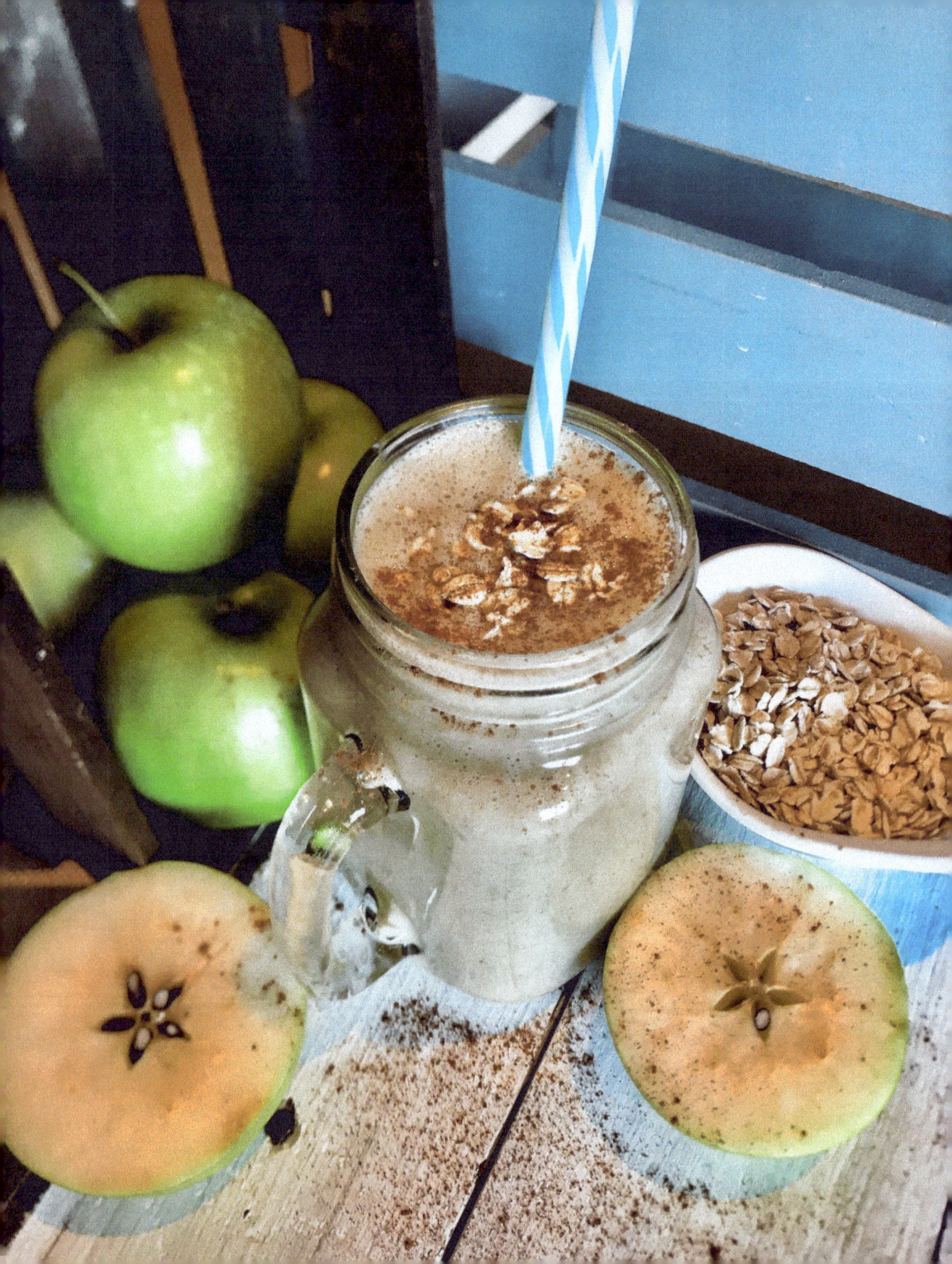

APPLE CRUMBLE SMOOTHIE

SERVES 2

2 Granny smith apples

3 tbsp organic, sugar free apple puree

1 tsp cinnamon

1 tbsp ground flaxseed

¼ cup of organic jumbo oats

2 tbsp local organic honey

unsweetened oat milk

Wash and roughly chop apples, removing the core & seeds

Place all ingredients in the nutri-bullet cup and fill to the max line with the oatmilk.

Blitz for 1 minute and serve.

Cinnamon helps balance blood sugar levels.

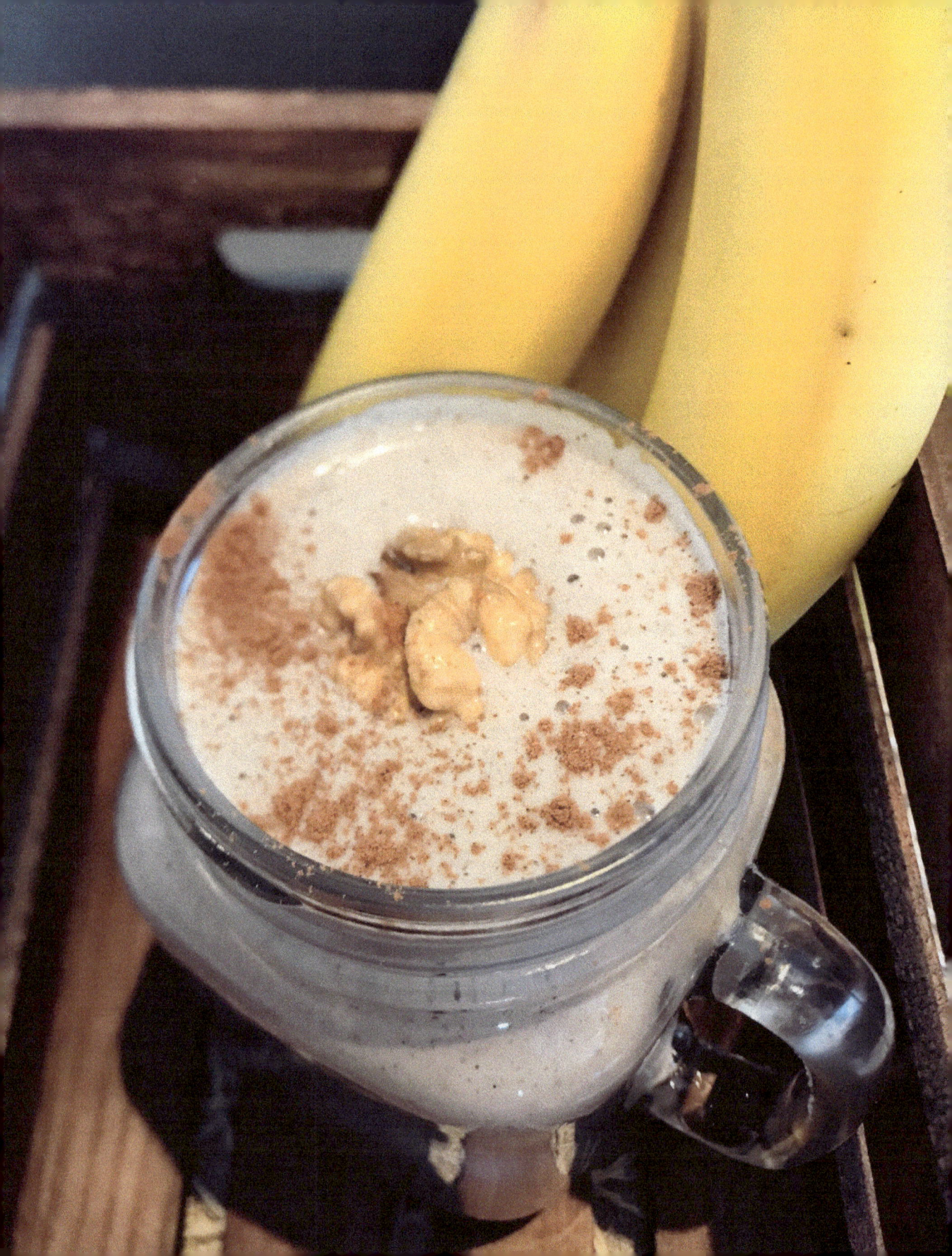

NUT BOOST SMOOTHIE

20 grams hazelnuts

20 grams almonds

20 grams brazil nuts

20 grams walnuts

20 grams pumpkin seeds

20 grams sunflower seeds

It's best to soak the above nuts & seeds in filtered water overnight. sieve and rinse before making the smoothie.

1 tbsp ground flaxseed

1 tsp cinnamon

1 tbsp organic local honey

1 banana

Oatmilk

Place the activated nuts and the other ingredients in the nutri-bullet cup and fill to the max line with the oatmilk.

Blitz for 1 minute and serve.

4 Brazil Nuts per day provide your daily recommended intake of Selenium, which is crucial to many bodily functions from mood to inflammation.

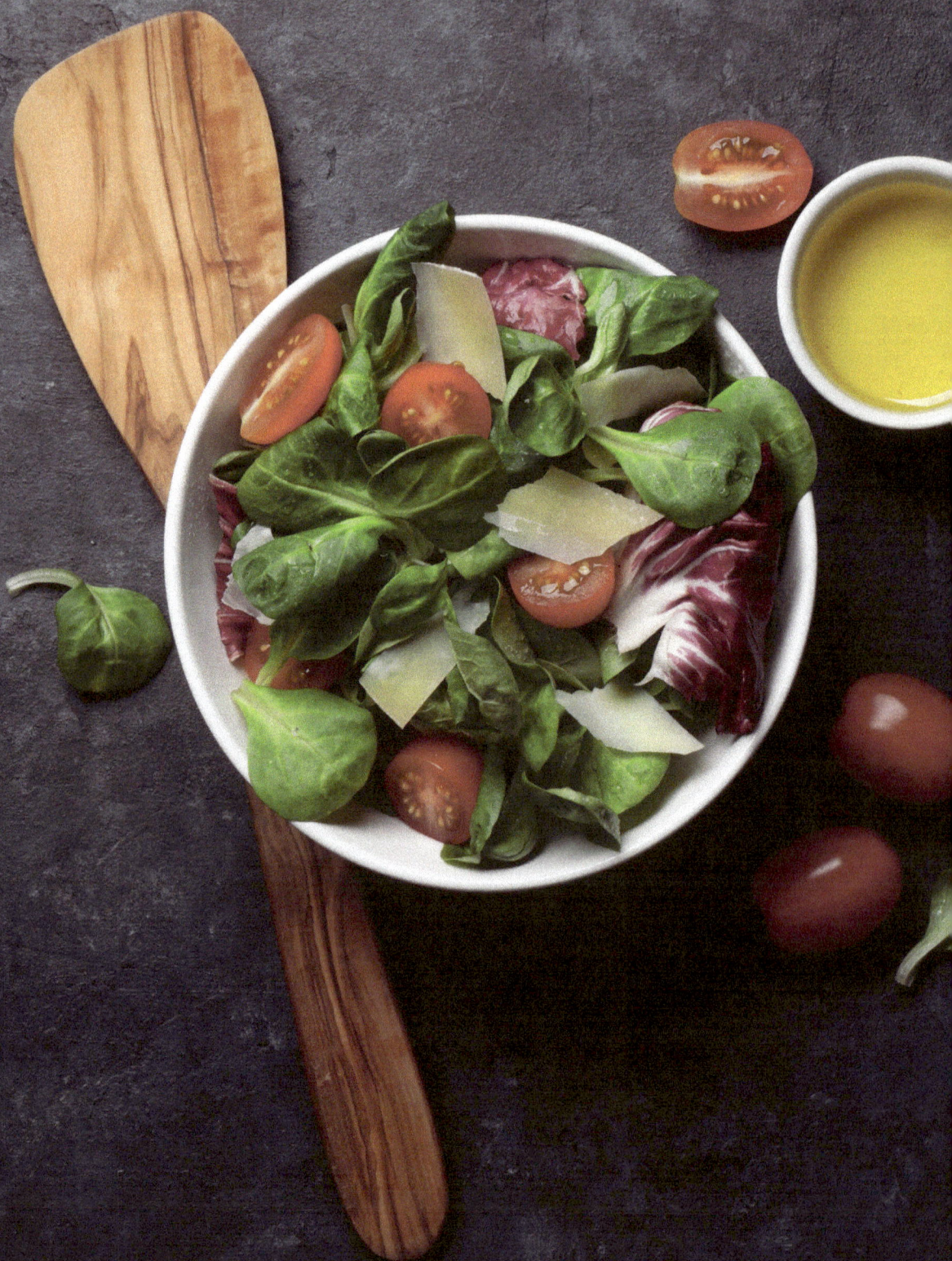

SERIOUS SALADS

Consuming more raw vegetables and fruit is
fundamental to good health. As we age, the amount
of enzymes we produce lessens, year after year.
Enzymes are important for a normal metabolism,
luckily, raw organic vegetables and fruits are packed
with enzymes, time to load up!

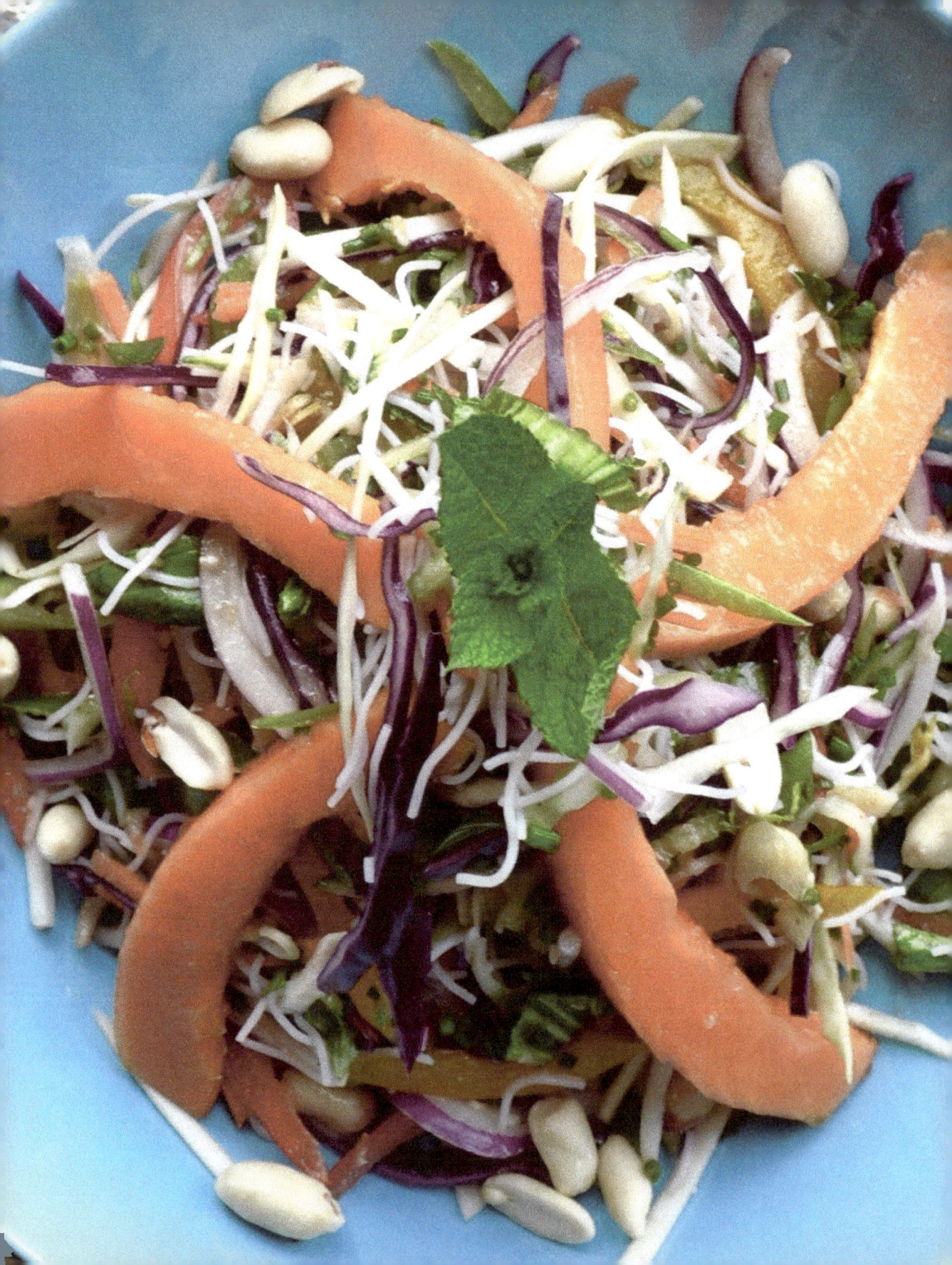

BANG BANG ASIAN RICE NOODLE SALAD

SERVES 2

50 grams shredded Red Cabbage

50 grams shredded White Cabbage

2 Spring Onions finely chopped

1 handful of Mange Tout finely sliced

¼ Cucumber shredded

1 small Carrot shredded

½ Red Pepper thinly sliced

½ Green Pepper thinly sliced

½ Yellow Pepper thinly sliced

1 Head of Bok choy finely chopped

½ Red Onion thinly sliced

½ cup of chopped Chives, Coriander and mint (save some for the dressing)

50 grams Beansprouts (washed and rinsed in salted water) alternatively use tinned beansprouts if pregnant or you have any health issues

50 grams Jumbo Peanuts

150 grams cooked Rice Noodles

1 Ripe Papaya, skinned, deseeded and sliced into thin wedges

FOR THE DRESSING

Mix the following ingredients in a bowl with a whisk

3 TBSP extra virgin organic Olive Oil

1 TBSP Apple Cider Vinegar (with the mother)

The juice of 1 Orange

The juice of 1 Lime

1 TBSP Sesame Oil

1 TBSP Sesame Seeds

1 TBSP Coconut & Peanut Butter

1 TBSP Tahini

2 TBSP Light Soy Sauce

½ Green Chilli finely sliced

½ Red Chilli finely sliced

1 TBSP Local Honey

The leftover herbs from above

Mix all the salad ingredients together in a large bowl, pour on the desired amount of dressing to just coat the salad.

Serve salad in bowls and garnish with papaya and some extra peanuts.

Papaya contains natural digestive enzymes.

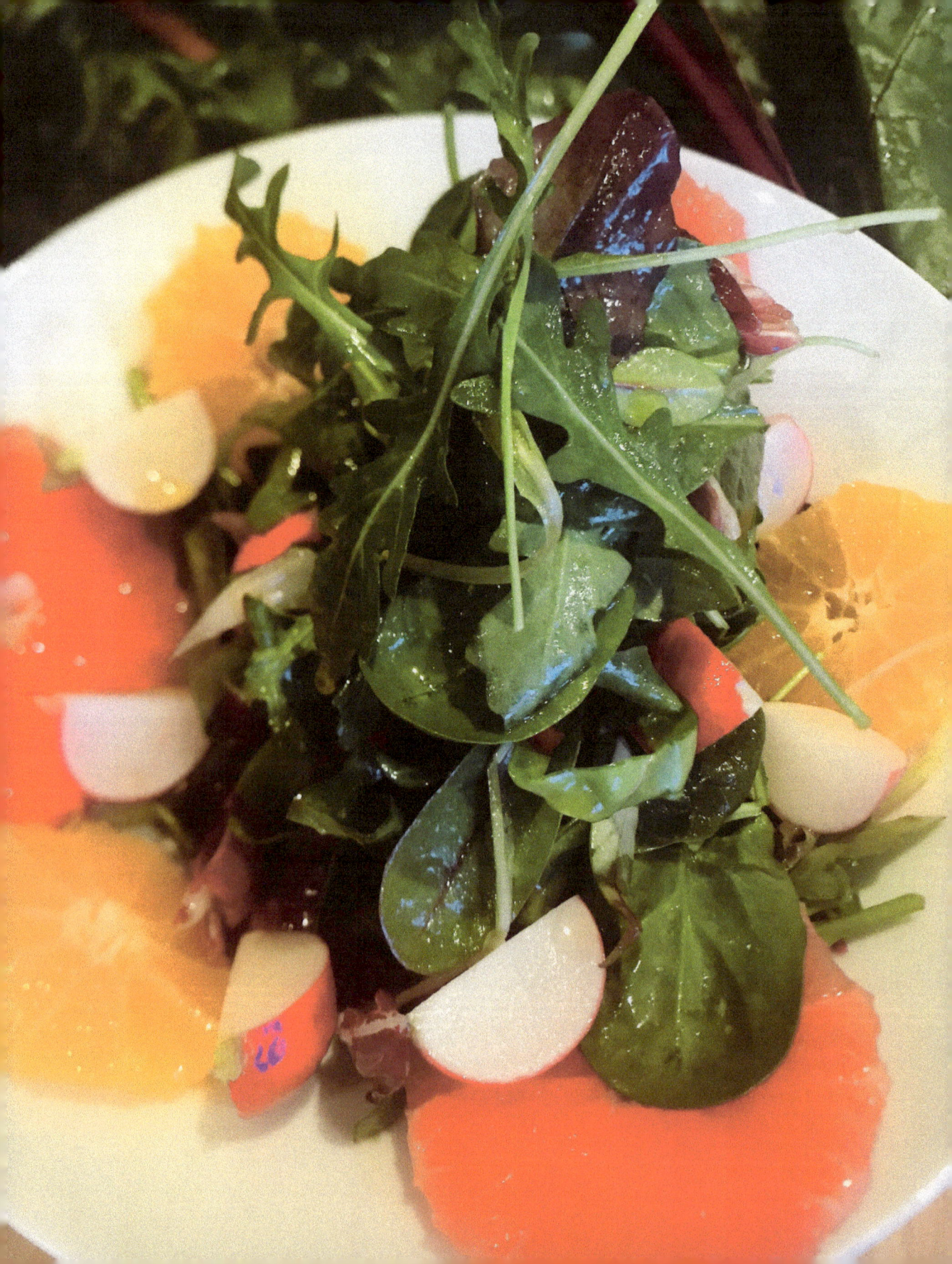

BITTER LEAF SALAD WITH CITRUS AND RADISH

SERVES 2

1 Ruby Grapefruit

1 Mandarin orange

4 Radishes

Selection of Bitter leaves

Red chard

Rainbow chard

Rocket

Radicchio

Baby spinach

Oakleaf

Endive

Chicory

Dressing, mix together the following

> 3 tbsp extra virgin organic olive oil
>
> 1 tbsp apple cider vinegar (with the mother)
>
> ½ tsp Dijon mustard
>
> ½ tsp organic local honey

Peel and slice citrus fruits into rounds, wash & cut radishes into small wedges. Wash and spin dry all leaves. Toss salad with desired amount of dressing and serve with radishes and citrus fruits.

Bitter leaves stimulate the production of digestive juices, such as saliva and bile.

EASY BUT POWERFUL KIMCHI

1 nappa Chinese cabbage

1 small daikon (Asian radish)

2 spring onions

1 thumb-size piece of ginger, peeled & finely chopped

4 cloves of garlic crushed

2 tbsp of ground Himalayan pink salt

4 tbsp of Korean red pepper flakes (gochugaru)

1 tbsp raw organic honey

60 mls of filtered water

Cut the cabbage into large chunks (remove any core). Place in a large mixing bowl and add the salt. Massage for 10 minutes with clean hands and leave for 1 hour with a plate on top to weigh it down.

Meanwhile, peel and cut the daikon into thin strips, finely chop the spring onions.

Make a paste with the gochugaru, honey and water by stirring together in a small dish.

After 1 hour, rinse the cabbage under cold running water and drain for 2 minutes. Now put on some disposable gloves and thoroughly mix all the ingredients together, including the paste. You are now ready to store your kimchi in sterilised jars with clasp lids. Leave to ferment for 3 days, before transferring to the fridge. Your kimchi is ready to eat, however, leaving it for a few more days will develop more flavour through natural fermentation.

Kimchi provides probiotics that help improve digestion.

CAPRESE SALAD

SERVES 2

2 large organic vine tomatoes

6 orange rapture tomatoes (or similar)

Fresh basil leaves

4 tsp Oat crème fraiche

4 tbsp organic extra virgin olive oil

freshly ground black pepper

Ground Himalayan salt

Wash and slice tomatoes and arrange on sharing plate along with basil leaves.

Dress with oat crème fraiche, drizzle olive oil and season to taste.

Including plenty of organic extra virgin olive oil in the diet can help with weight loss, controlling excess insulin.

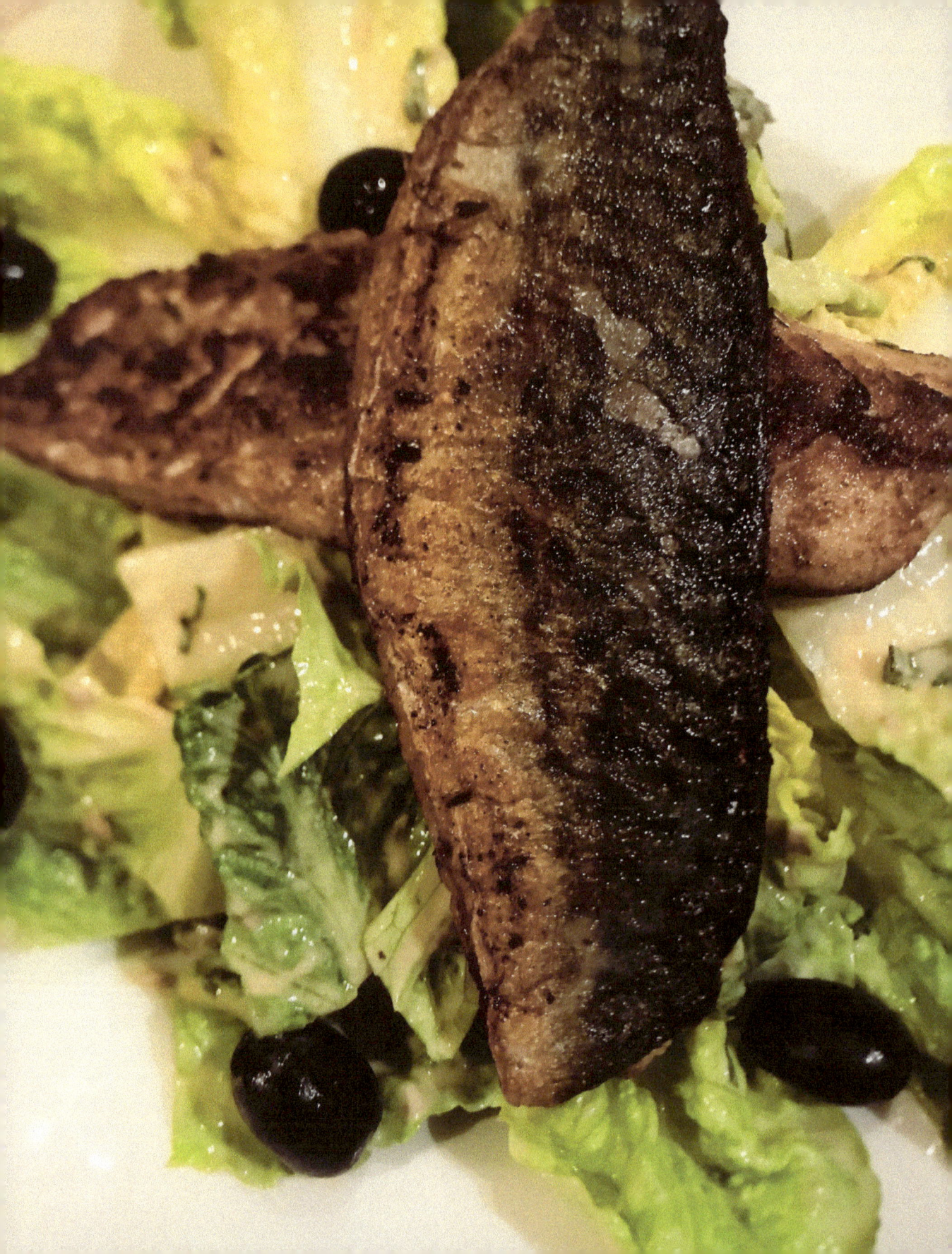

CAJUN SPICED MACKEREL
CAESAR SALAD

SERVES 2

2 fresh mackerel fillets (deboned) lightly seasoned with cajun spice and lightly rubbed with olive oil

1 large romaine lettuce washed and chopped

For the dressing thoroughly mix the following (this version of a Caesar dressing really packs a punch of flavour, compensating for heavy parmesan and mayo).

2 tbsp finely chopped basil

3 tbsp organic extra virgin olive oil

10 anchovy fillets very finely chopped

the juice of 1 whole lemon

2 tbsp Worcestershire sauce

1 tsp Tabasco sauce

2 heaped tbsp. oat crème fraiche

freshly ground pepper

Once you have everything prepared, pan fry the fish for 2.5 mins each side approx. in a hot non-stick frying pan, transfer to a plate to rest.

Toss the romaine lettuce with the desired amount of dressing, serve with fish on top and garnish with some black olives (optional).

Mackerel is an omega-3 powerhouse, it supports heart and brain health. It is also a great source of vitamin B12 which supports energy levels.

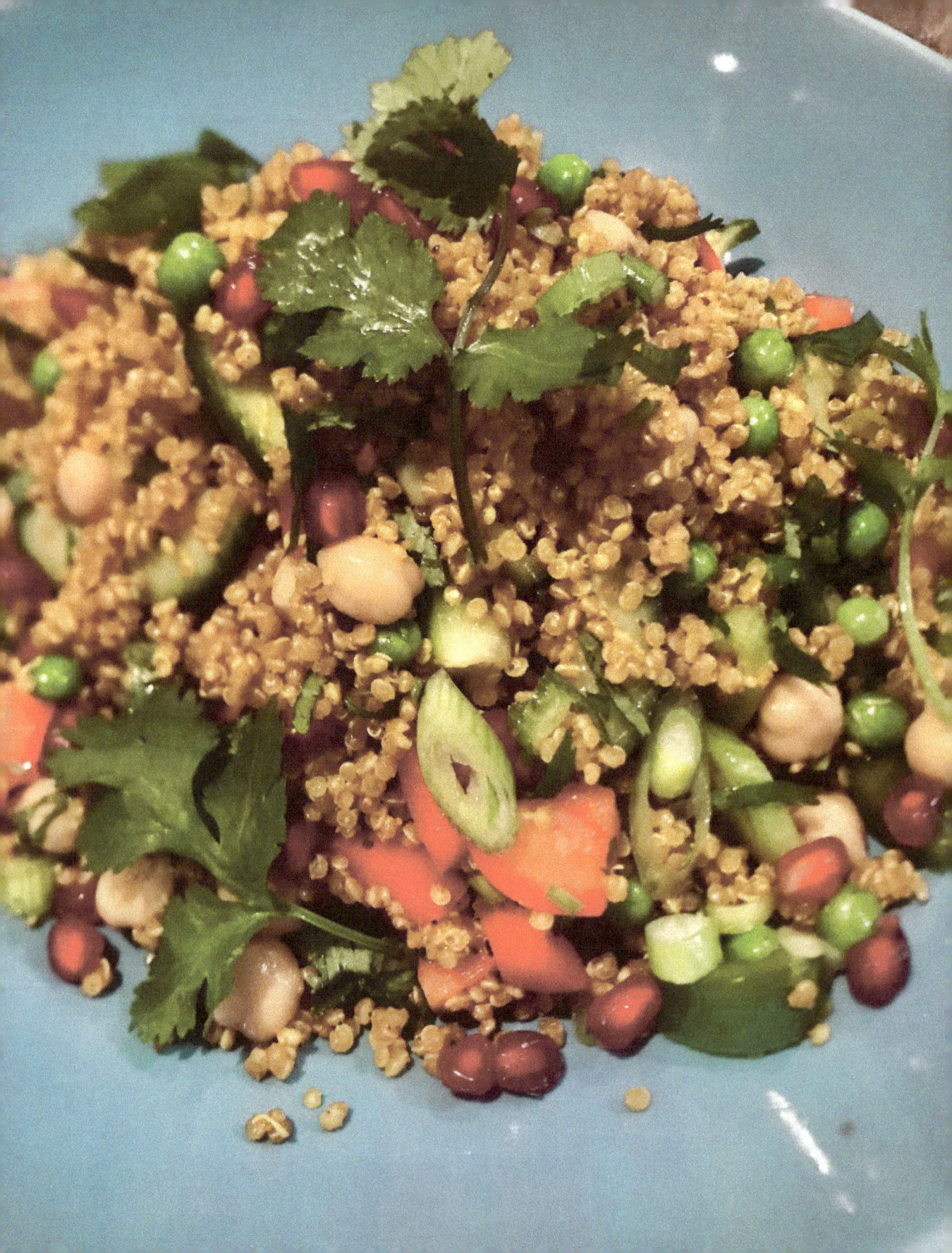

CURRIED QUINOA TABOULLEH SALAD

SERVES 2

1 cup quinoa

2 cups boiling water

1 organic vegetable stock cube

1 heaped tsp of madras curry paste

1 tsp turmeric powder

75 grams cooked and rinsed chickpeas

2 heaped tbsp. chopped coriander

2 spring onions chopped

1 cup of diced green and red pepper

½ cup of frozen peas defrosted

1 cup of sliced cucumber

50 grams pomegranate seeds

2 tbsp organic extra virgin olive oil

Himalayan salt

Place all the above ingredients in a small saucepan, boil on a high heat for 10-12 mins, stirring regularly with a whisk. Remove from the heat and put a lid on the pot to allow the quinoa to finish cooking in its own residual heat, this should take a further 10 mins. Transfer to a large plate and allow to cool.

Once the quinoa is cooled, place in a mixing bowl with all the above ingredients, season to taste with the Himalayan salt.

Mix well and serve with extra pomegranate seeds.

Quinoa is a complete source of protein, it contains all nine essential amino acids, important for growth and repair.

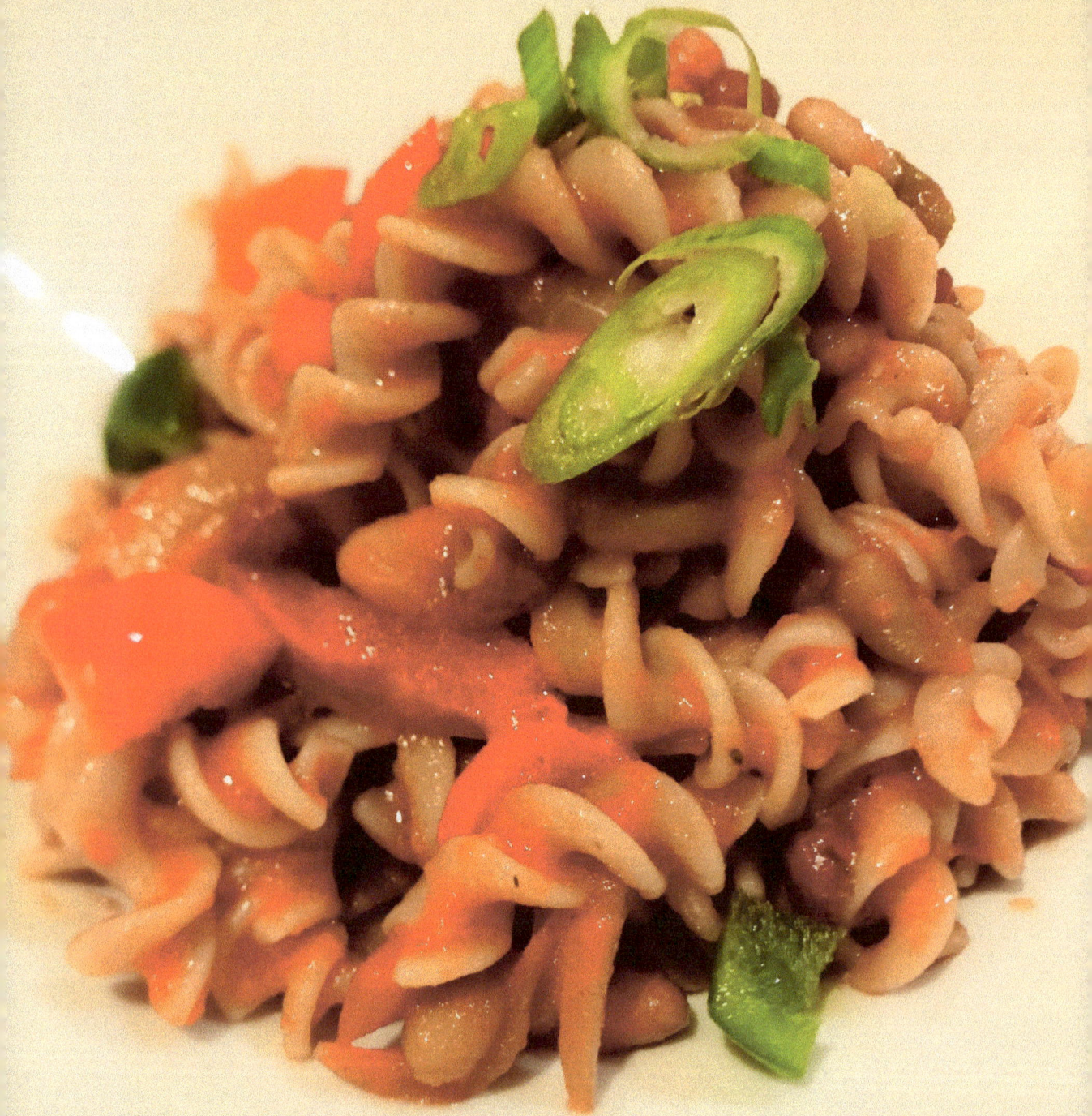

MEXICAN BEAN RICE PASTA SALAD

SERVES 4

1 red pepper sliced

1 green pepper sliced

2 small onions peeled and sliced

2 garlic cloves crushed

1 tbsp fajita spice

70 grams tomato puree

500 grams tomato passata

2 × 400 gram tins of mixed beans rinsed

freshly ground black pepper

Ground Himalayan salt

1tbsp organic extra virgin olive oil

1 250 gram bag of brown rice pasta

2 tbsp of sriracha chilli sauce

Preheat a large non-stick frying pan, add olive oil and fry peppers, onions and garlic for 3 mins. Add a splash of boiling water to create some steam, sprinkle in the fajita spice and add tomato puree. Stir and cook for 2 minutes, then add the passata and beans. Continue to cook for a further 10 minutes, stirring regularly. Remove from the heat and allow to cool.

Cook the pasta in boiling salted water for 9 mins approx. (follow instructions on pack, and cool down rapidly under cold water, strain and leave to one side.)

Once everything is cooled, mix together the beans, pasta and sriracha sauce in a large mixing bowl and season with Himalayan salt to taste.

Brown rice pasta is a great gluten free alternative to conventional wheat pasta, it is nutrient dense and promotes a healthy gut.

77

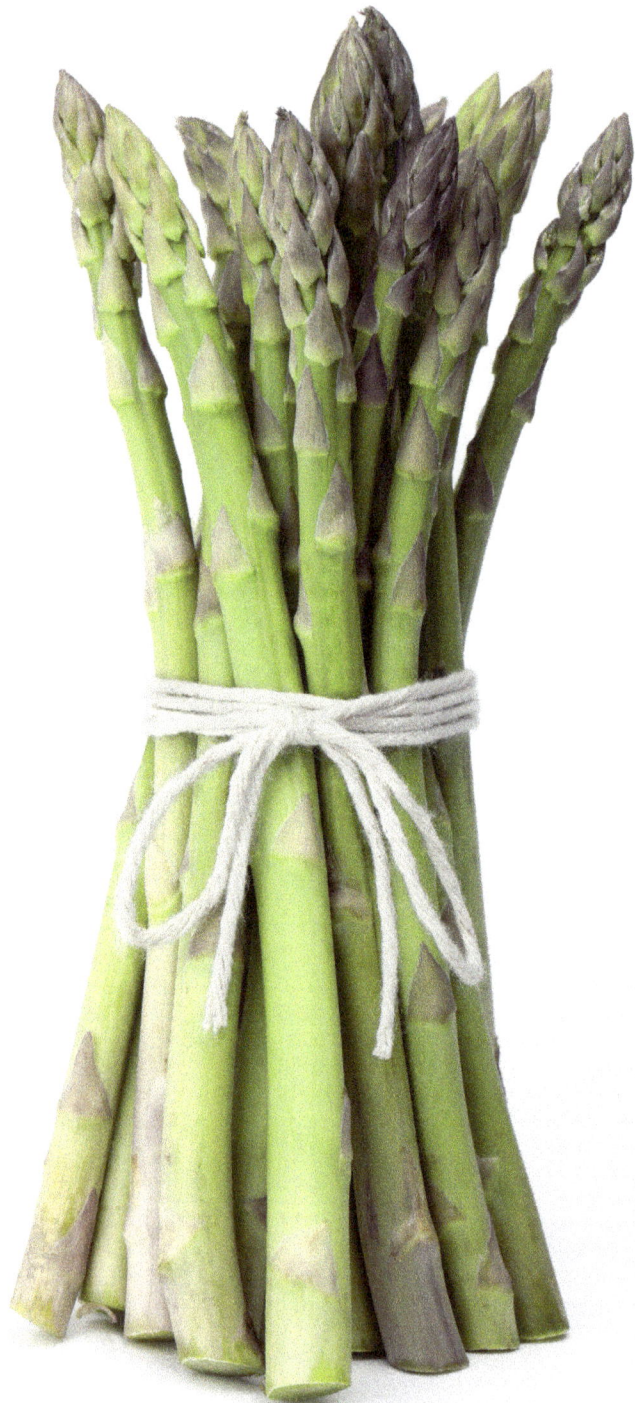

SIMPLE NICOISE SALAD

SERVES 2

50 grams fine green beans (trimmed)

50 grams tender stem broccoli

50 grams asparagus

1 large vine tomato cut into wedges

4 baby potatoes

4 boiled organic eggs

10 black olives (pitted)

10 anchovy fillets

30 grams sweetcorn (frozen or canned)

4 radishes cut into wedges

½ romaine lettuce sliced

3 tbsp organic extra virgin olive oil

1 tbsp apple cider vinegar(with mother)

½ tsp Dijon mustard

½ tsp organic local honey

ground Himalayan salt

Freshly ground black pepper

Blanch and refresh the beans, broccoli and asparagus in boiling salted water then plunge into ice water and drain. Cut the potatoes into wedges and air-fry for 15 minutes. Boil the eggs for 5 minutes, cool, peel and cut the eggs in half.

Mix together the olive oil, acv, mustard & honey for the dressing, seasoning to taste.

In a large mixing bowl bring all the ingredients together and dress with vinaigrette holding back the eggs and anchovies to arrange on top.

Asparagus is a great source of stress busting B vitamins.

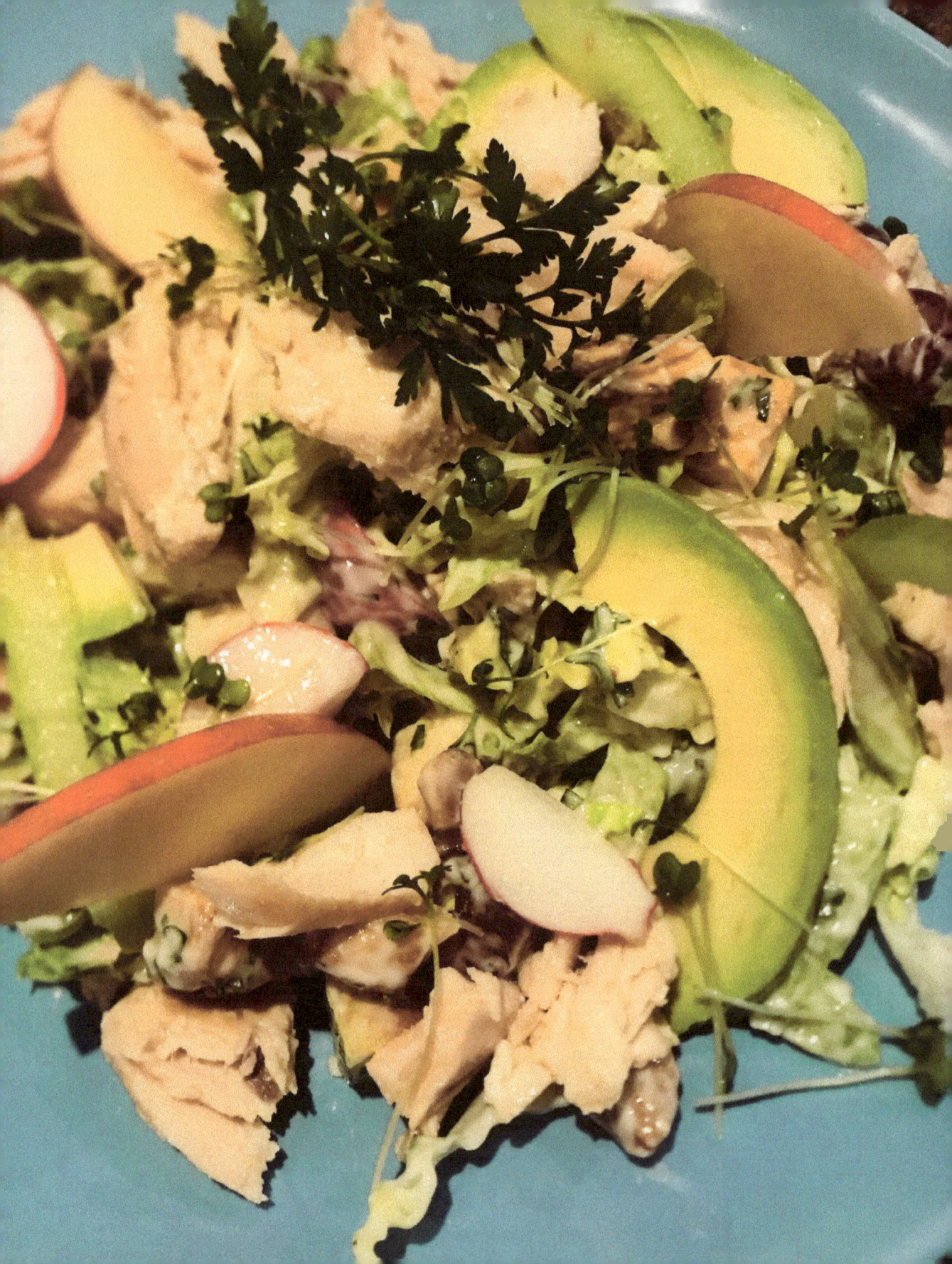

WILD ALASKAN SALMON WALDORF SALAD

SERVES 2

200 grams of wild Alaskan salmon or local wild salmon (skinless & boneless)

1 sweet potato

2 ribs of celery sliced

1 red apple cored and diced

20 walnut halves (soaked in water overnight)

½ an avocado sliced

20 mixed seedless grapes

½ a romaine lettuce, washed & sliced

2 heaped tbsp. oat crème fraiche

juice of half a lemon

2 tbsp chopped Italian parsley

Ground Himalayan salt

2 tbsp organic extra virgin olive oil

Freshly ground black pepper

Season the salmon and roast in a hot oven (180 °C) for 12 minutes approx. Allow to rest and cool. Once cool, flake the salmon.

Cut the sweet potato into small chunks and air-fry for 15 minutes and allow to cool.

Mix together the oat crème fraiche, lemon juice, parsley & olive oil and season to taste.

In a large mixing bowl, toss together all the ingredients except the salmon, and stir in the dressing. Serve and arrange the flaked salmon on top and around.

Grapes contain a variety of antioxidants which contribute to glowing skin, heart health and prevention of oxidative stress.

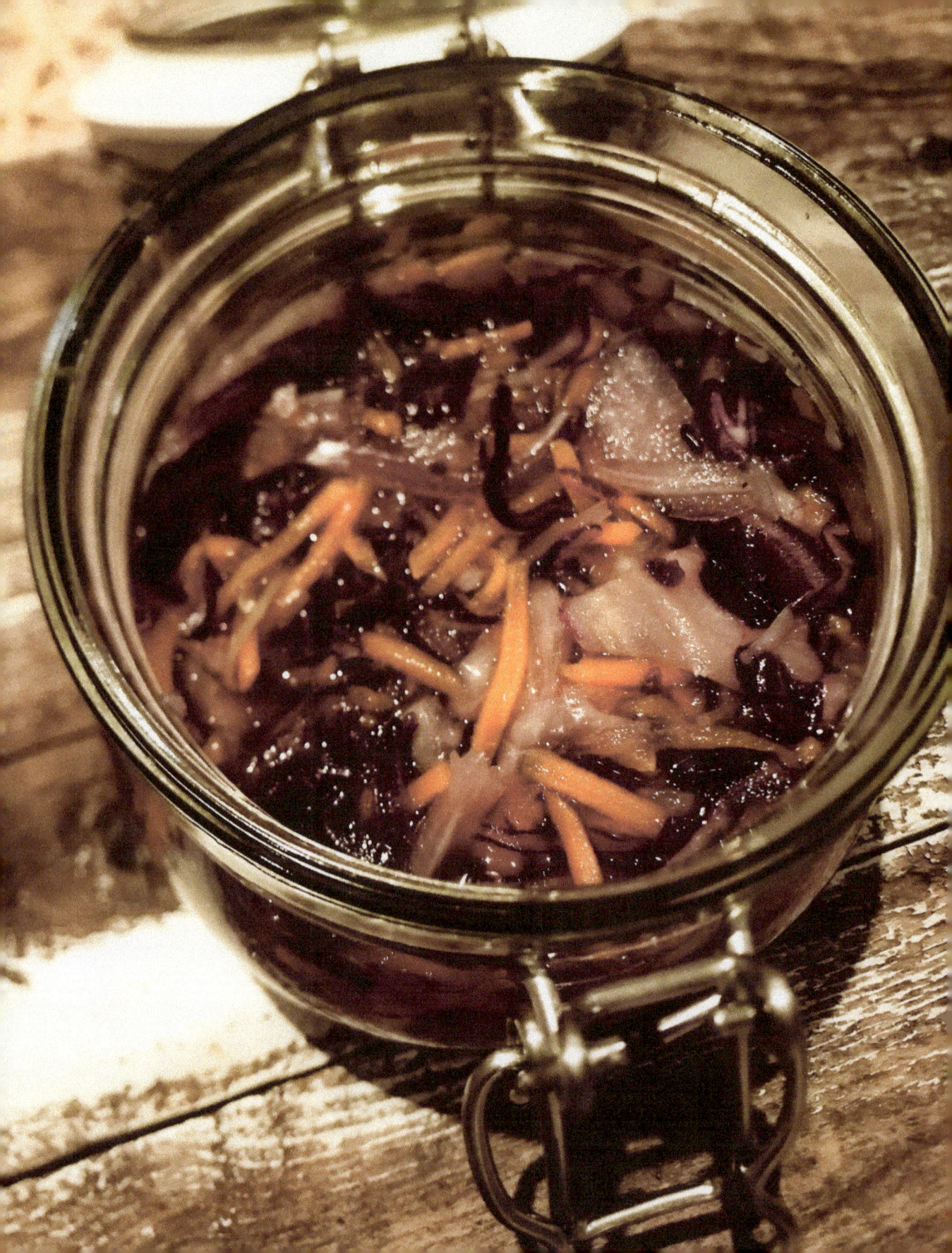

SAUERKRAUT SALAD

250 grams of finely sliced white cabbage

250 grams of finely slices red cabbage

1 small carrot, peeled & grated

½ of a small red onion finely sliced

1 tbsp of ground Himalayan pink salt

Place all ingredients in a mixing bowl. With clean hands, scrunch the vegetables for a good 10 minutes, this speeds up the liquid being extracted.

Put the sauerkraut in a sterile glass jar with clasp lid, ensuring that the veg is fully submerged in the liquid (if necessary you can weigh down the sauerkraut with a piece of grease proof paper and a small weight).

Leave to ferment in a cool area for 3 days, before transferring to the fridge for at least another 4 days before consuming (thus allowing the flavour to develop).

Tip – each day after making, be sure to open the clasp lid to release any pressure that may build up, and close again.

Sauerkraut supports healthy gut flora.

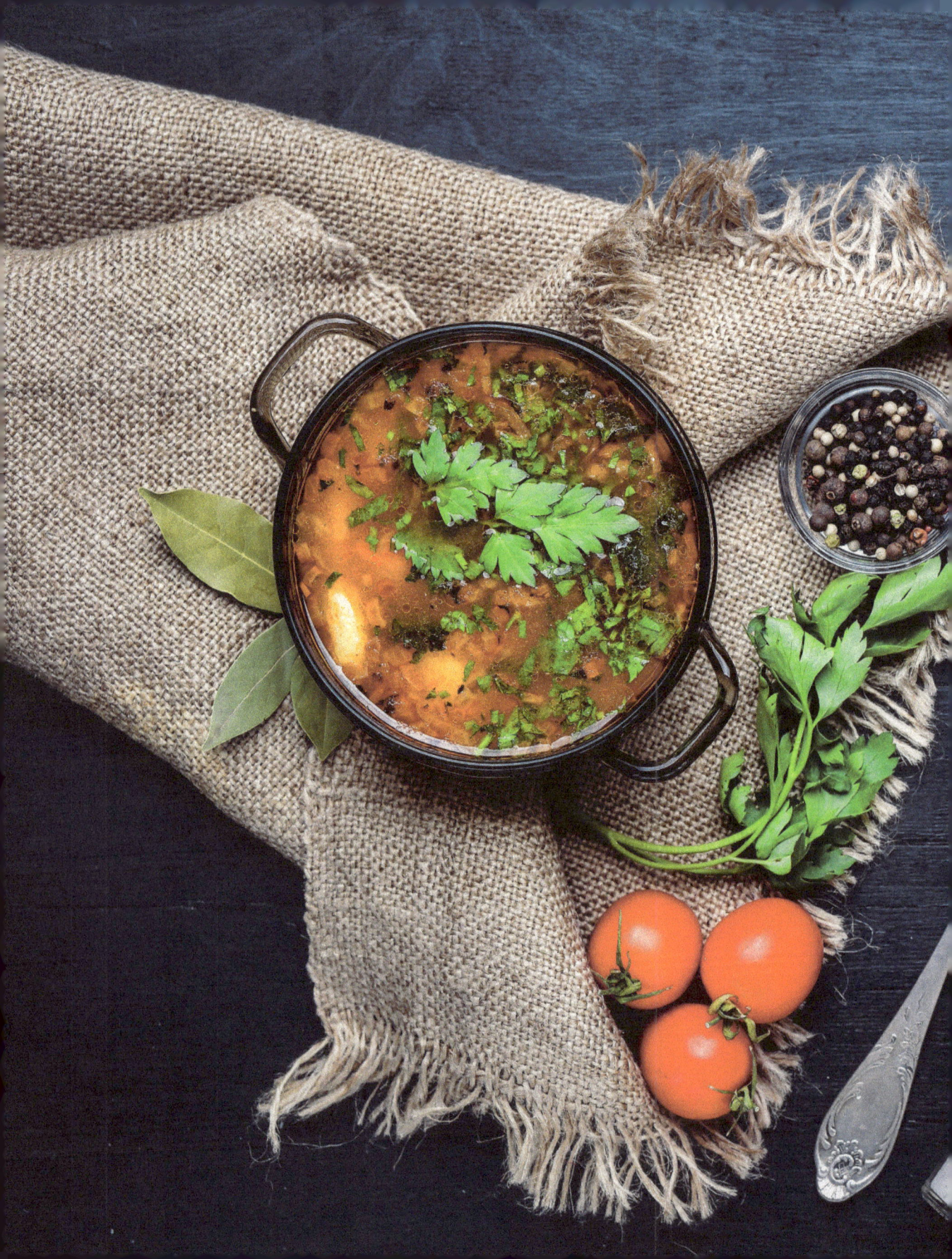

SOUPS
DE
JOUR

Nothing beats a soothing, comforting bowl of soup.
Each of the following recipes are easy digested and
promote good gut health.

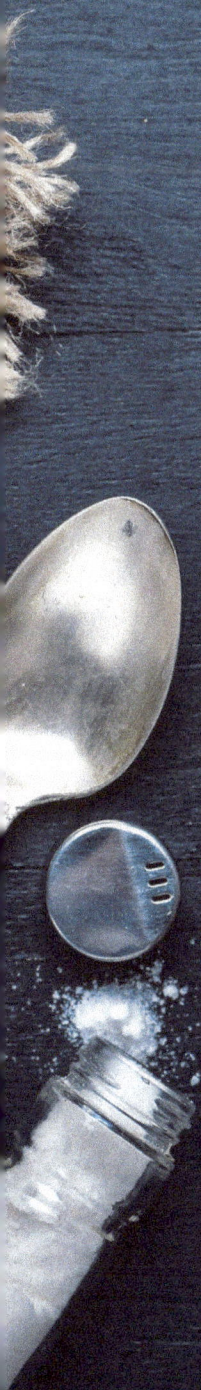

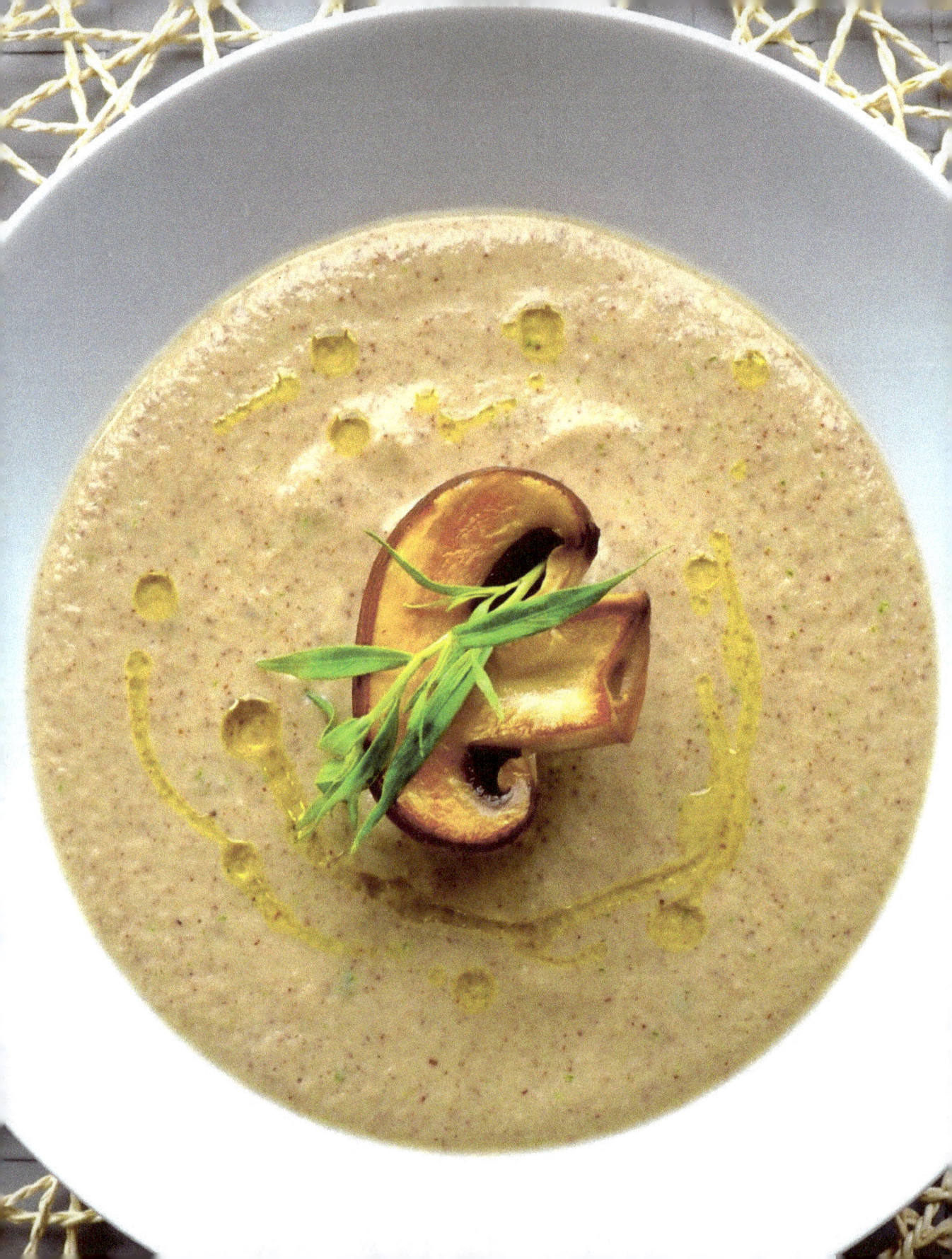

MIXED MUSHROOM, ALMOND & TARRAGON SOUP

SERVES 2

1 TSP extra virgin organic Olive oil

1 Small Onion

2 Cloves Garlic

200 Grams Chestnut Mushrooms

200 Grams White Mushrooms

1 (organic) vegetable Stock cube

2 TBSP chopped Tarragon Leaves

1 heaped TBSP Almond butter

1 Pint (568 mls) hot water

ground Himalayan Pink Salt

freshly ground Black Pepper

Roughly chop onion, Mushrooms and garlic and sauté in a medium stainless steel saucepan with the olive oil, add stock cube, hot water and tarragon.

Bring to boil and simmer for 10 minutes.

Add almond butter and blend using a handheld stick blender until silky smooth.

Season to taste with Himalayan salt and freshly ground black pepper.

Adjust consistency with a little hot water if the soup is too thick.

Mushrooms are a good source of vitamin D which supports immune function, they are also known to have anti-inflammatory and antibacterial effects.

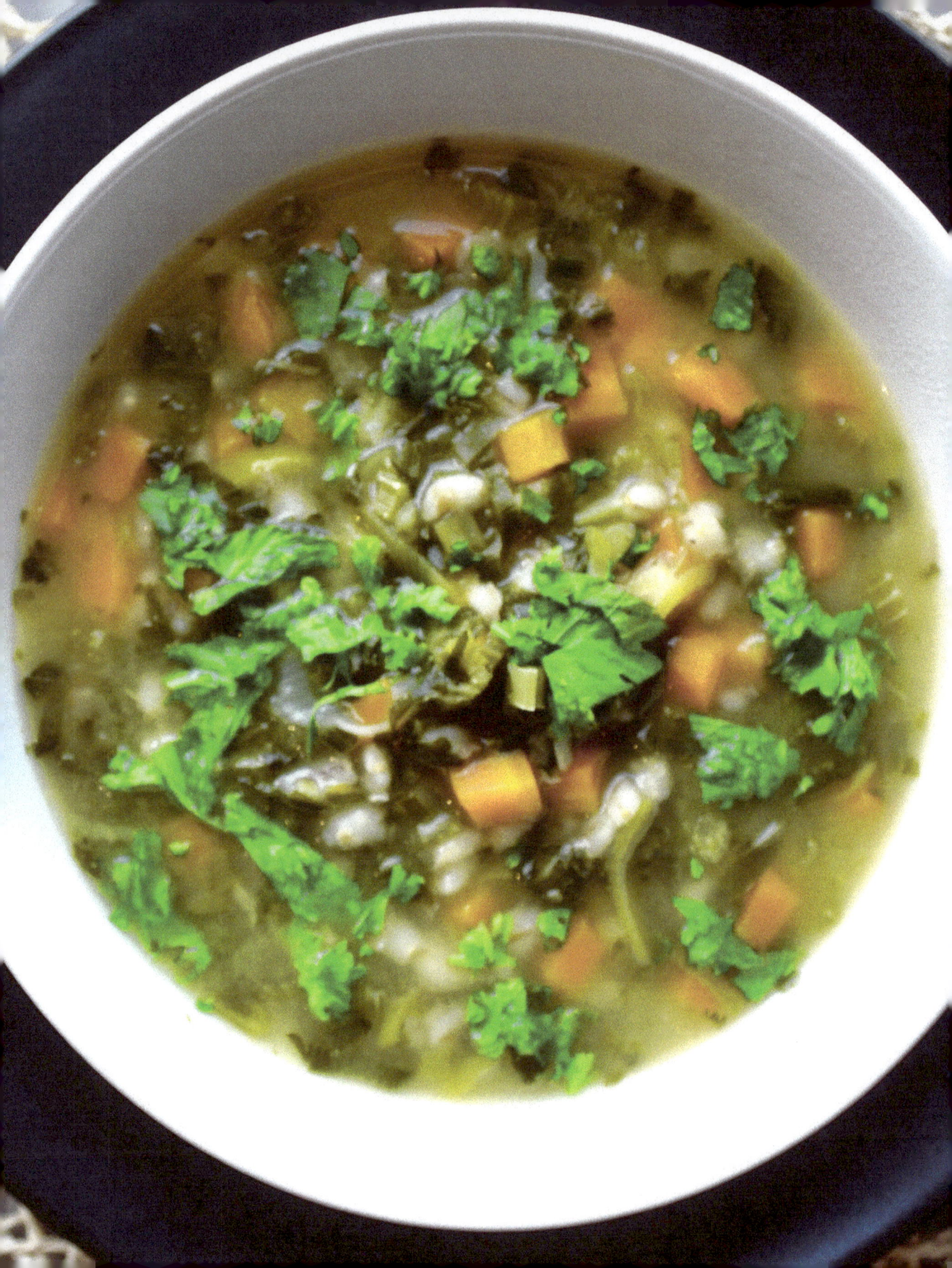

TRADITIONAL (NORTHERN IRISH) VEGETABLE BROTH

SERVES 4-6

100 Grams Pearl Barley (contains gluten)

2 Large Carrots

2 Small Soup Leeks or 1 large normal Leek

1 Large Bunch of Curly Parsley

1 Large Bunch of Soup Celery or 1 Head of Table Celery

2 Organic Vegetable Stock Cubes

1.5 Litres of Hot Water

Ground Himalayan Pink Salt

Freshly Ground Black Pepper

Steep barley in cold water for 2 hours or overnight in a large stainless steel saucepan.

Peel and chop carrots into small dice.

Roughly chop celery, leeks and parsley and rinse with cold water to remove any soil.

Rinse the barley well with cold water through a sieve and return to pan, cover with cold water and place pan on the stove, bring to the boil, reduce heat and simmer for 15 minutes.

Rinse the barley again with hot water from the kettle this time through a sieve (this removes a lot of the starchy gluten).

Return the barley to a clean saucepan with the carrots and 750 mls of hot water. Place on the stove on a high heat, bring to the boil, reduce heat and simmer for 10 mins.

Add the organic vegetable stock cubes and the celery, leeks and parsley, pour in the remaining 750 mls of hot water, stir well.

Turn the heat up and bring to the boil. Reduce heat and simmer for 20 minutes.

Season the broth with Himalayan pink salt and black pepper to taste.

Parsley supports healthy kidneys and bladder.

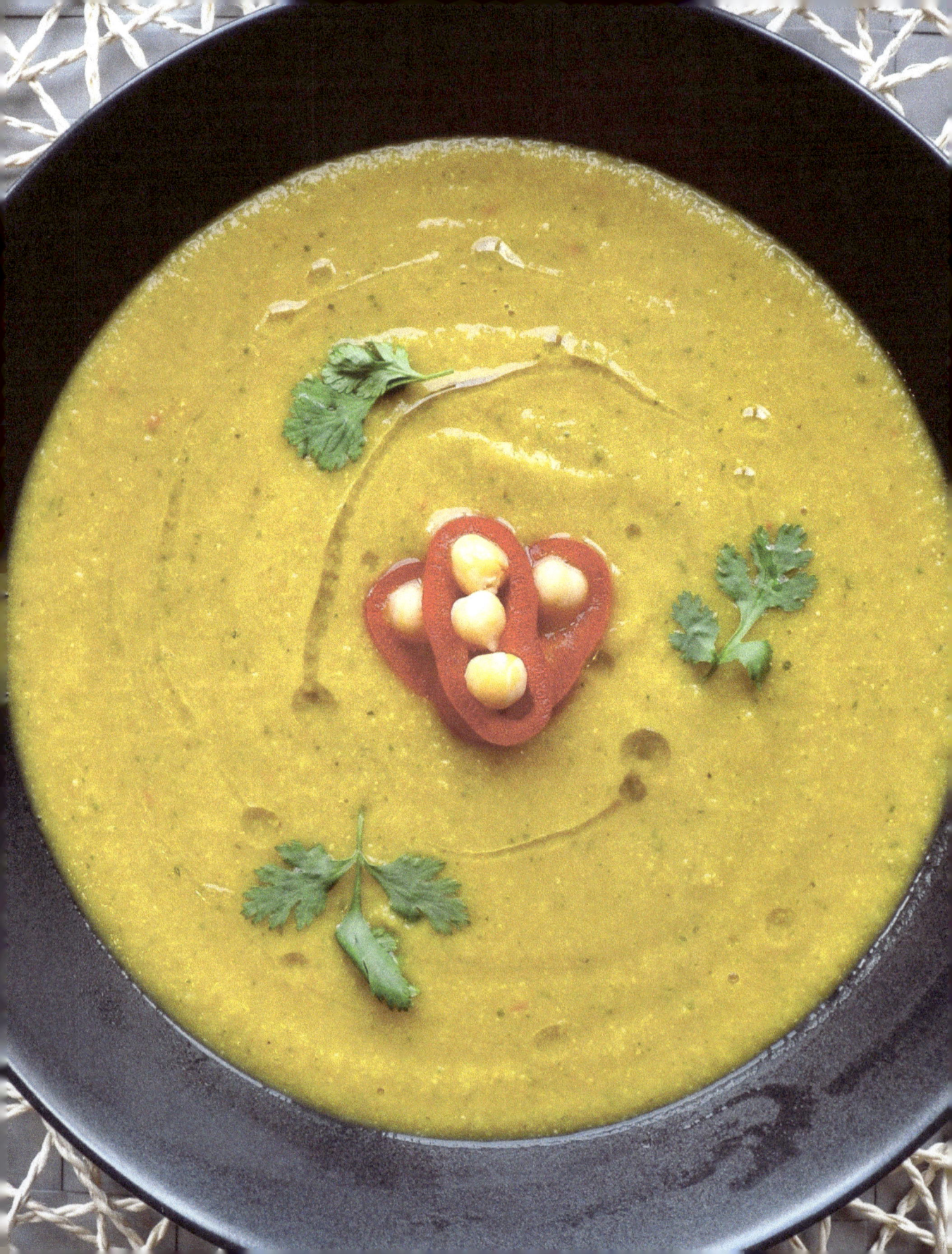

CHICKPEA, CHILLI AND CORIANDER SOUP

SERVES 4

1 Small White Onion

1 Medium Carrot

1 Rib of Celery

½ Red Chilli (seeds removed)

4 Cloves Garlic

1 Small Bunch Coriander

1 TSP Extra Virgin Organic Olive Oil

2 × 400 Gram Cans of Chickpeas (drained and rinsed)

1 Litre Hot Water

1 Organic Vegetable Stock Cube

Ground Himalayan Pink Salt

Freshly Ground Black pepper

Peel and roughly chop onion, carrot and garlic, wash celery and roughly chop also.

Roughly chop the chilli and coriander stocks (save leaves to last).

Place a medium stainless steel saucepan on the cooker on a medium heat. Add the olive oil, onion, carrot, celery, garlic, chilli and coriander stocks and sauté for 5 minutes.

Add chickpeas, hot water and stock cube to the pan, bring to the boil and then simmer for 30 minutes.

Liquidise the soup with a handheld stick blender.

Season to taste with freshly ground black pepper and Himalayan pink salt.

Adjust the consistency of the soup with a little hot water if necessary.

Chickpeas increase satiety and can aid in weight loss.

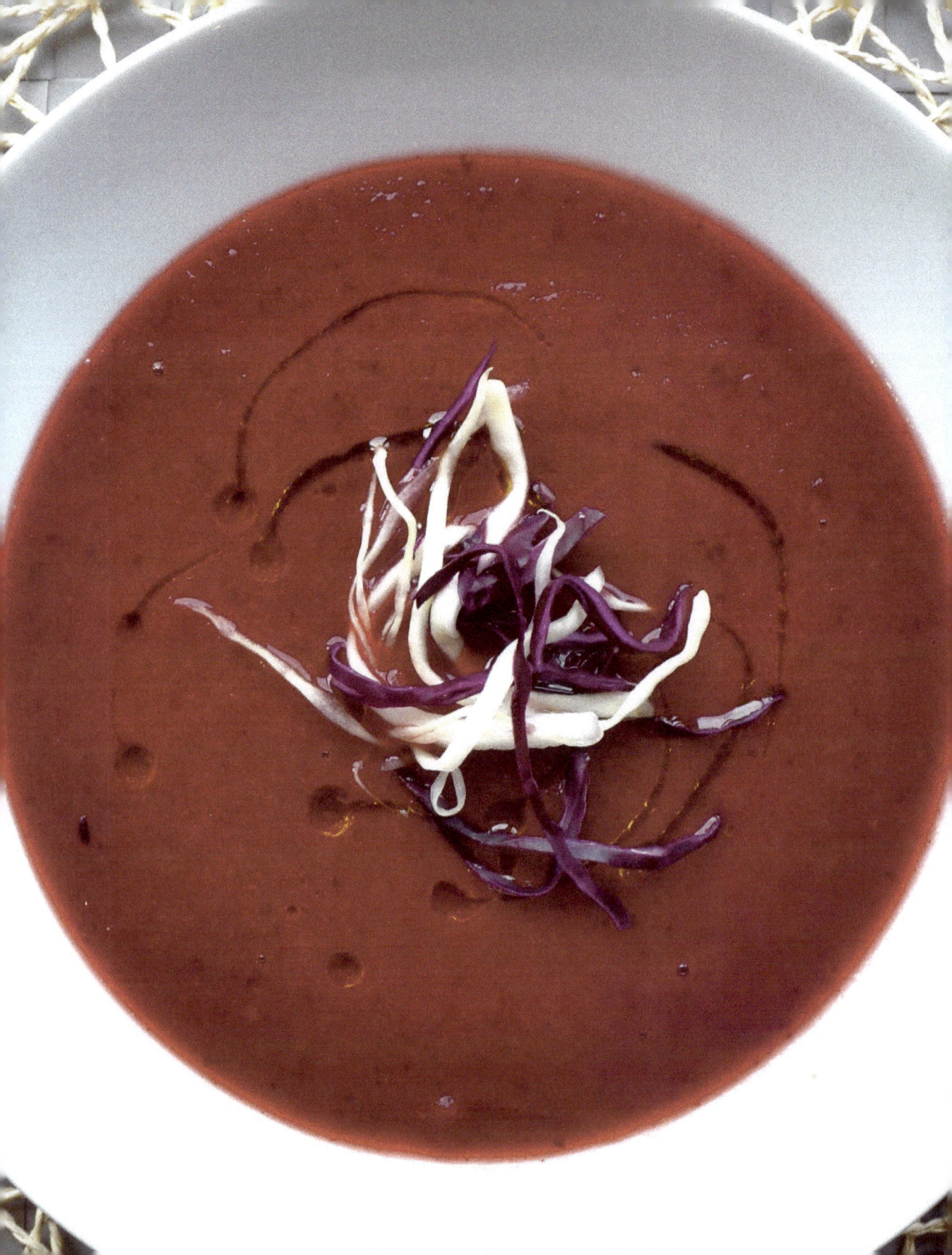

RED CABBAGE, BEETROOT, APPLE AND KIDNEY BEAN SOUP

SERVES 4

1 Small Onion

1 Rib of Celery

1 Medium Carrot

1 Clove of Garlic

1 Tsp extra virgin organic Olive Oil

¼ of a Small Red Cabbage

150 Grams Cooked Beetroot

1 Granny Smith Apple

100 Grams Cooked Rinsed Kidney Beans (canned is fine)

1 Organic Vegetable Stock Cube

750 mls hot water

Ground Himalayan Pink salt

Freshly Ground Black pepper

Peel and roughly chop onion, carrot, garlic and apple (remove core).

Wash celery and chop, roughly chop cabbage and beetroot.

Place a large stainless steel saucepan on the cooker on a medium heat. Add olive oil, onion, celery, carrot, garlic, apple, cabbage and beetroot, sauté for 10 minutes whilst stirring occasionally.

Add kidney beans, stock cube and hot water.

Bring to the boil, turn heat down to medium, put a lid on and simmer for 1 hour.

Check that all the vegetables are tender with a small knife and liquidise with a handheld stick blender.

Season to taste with freshly ground black pepper and Himalayan pink salt.

Adjust consistency of the soup with a little hot water if necessary.

Red cabbage supports stomach health. It also fights free radical damage to skin.

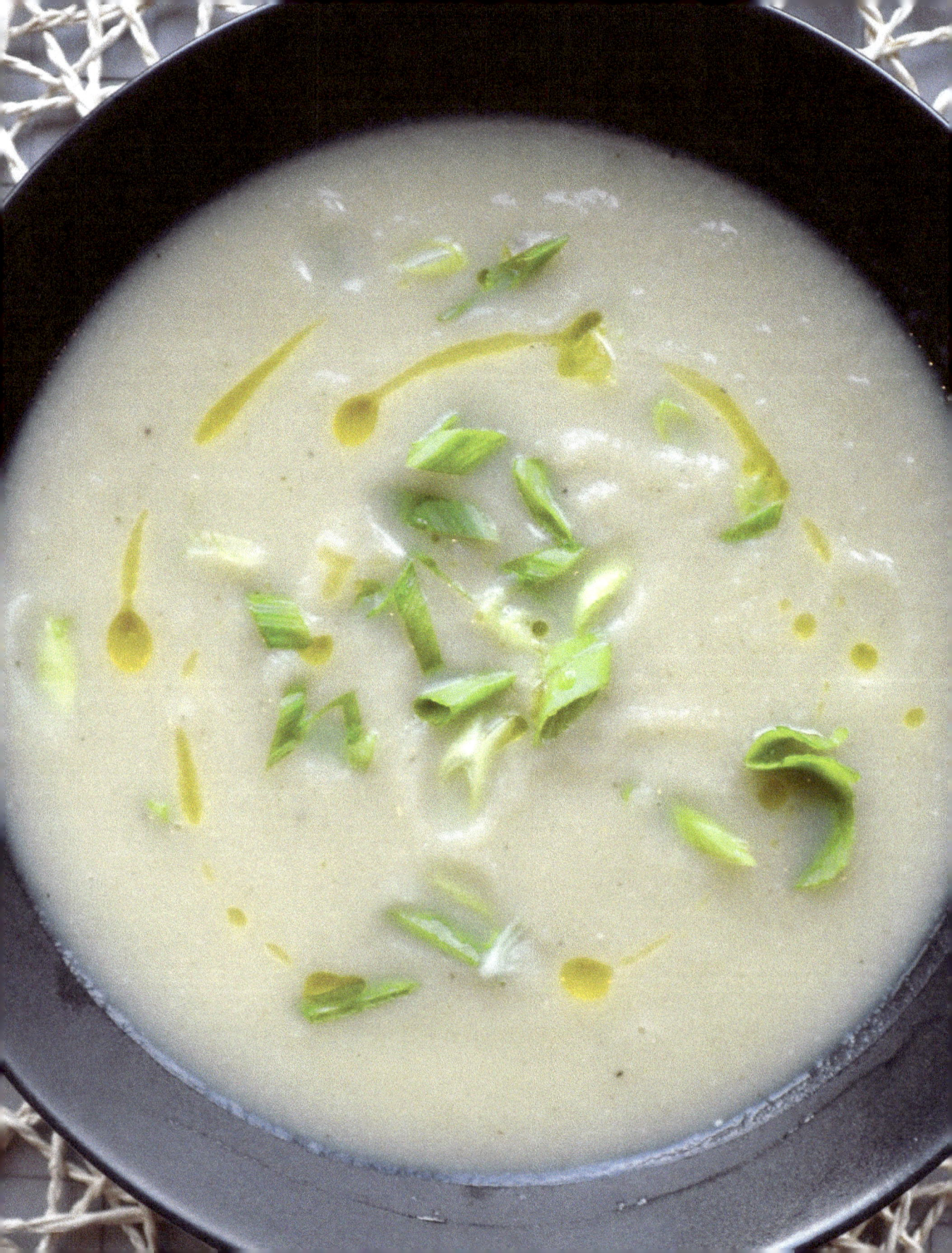

CELERIAC, ONION AND THYME SOUP

SERVES 4

1 TBSP Extra Virgin Organic Olive Oil

2 Small Onions

1 Celeriac

2 Cloves of Garlic

2 TBSP Chopped Fresh Thyme Leaves

1 Litre of Hot Water

1 Organic Vegetable Stock Cube

2 Spring Onions

Himalayan Pink Salt

Black Pepper

Peel and roughly chop onions, celeriac and garlic.

Place a large stainless steel saucepan on a medium heat, add olive oil, onions, celeriac, garlic and thyme. Sauté for 5 minutes, whilst stirring to prevent colouring the vegetables.

Pour in the hot water and add the stock cube, turn the heat up and bring to the boil. Reduce heat, lid on and simmer for 30 minutes until all the ingredients are tender.

Liquidise the soup with a handheld stick blender, season with freshly ground black pepper and Himalayan pink salt.

Adjust consistency of the soup with a little extra hot water if necessary.

Wash and finely chop spring onions for garnish.

Celeriac helps bone density and prevents osteoporosis due to high levels of vitamin K.

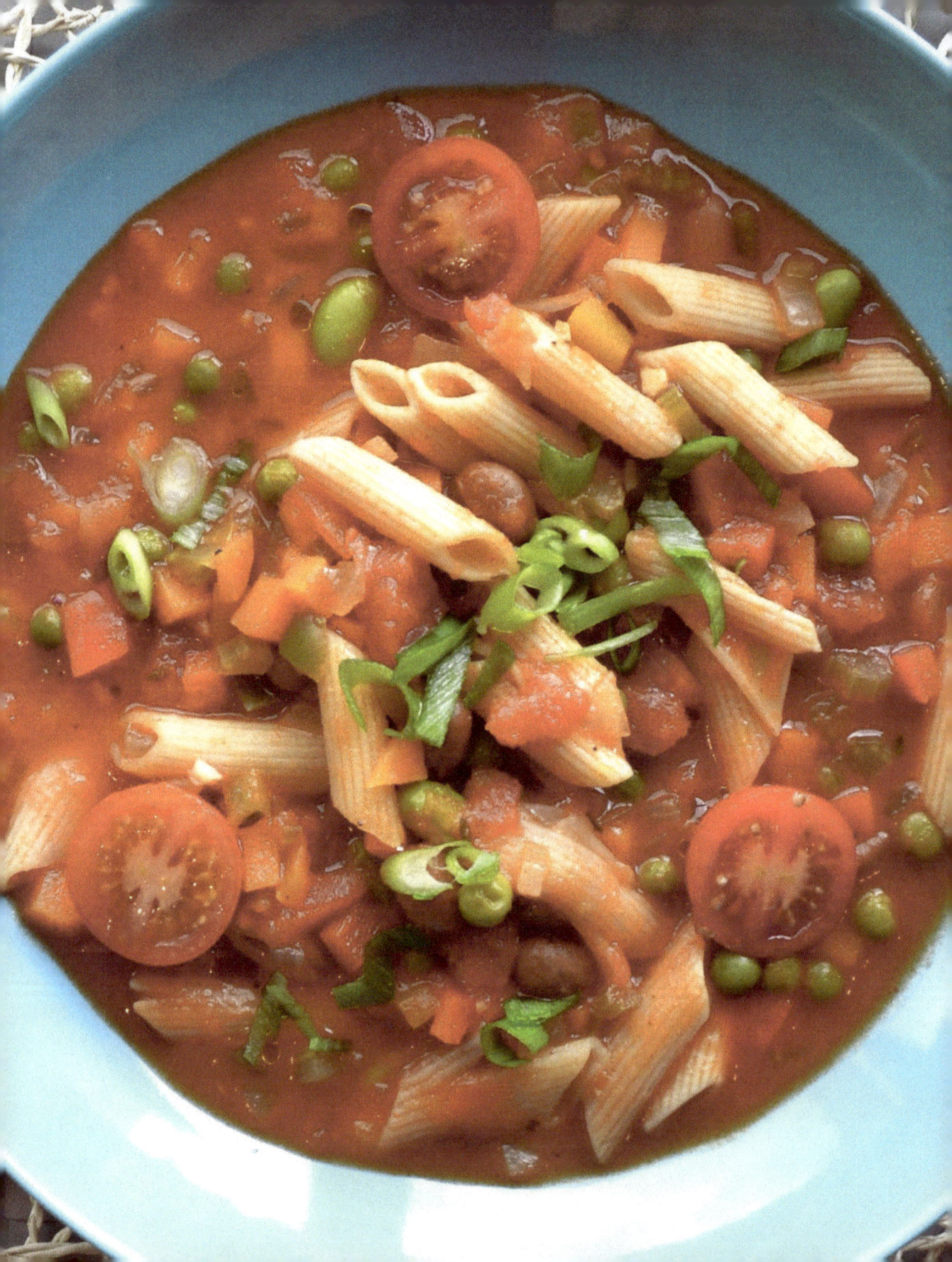

MEXICAN MINESTRONE

SERVES 4

100 Grams Spelt Penne Pasta (Alternative: Whole Wheat Penne or Brown Rice fusilli Pasta)

1 TBSP Extra Virgin Organic Olive Oil

1 Small Onion

1 Small Carrot

1 Rib Of Celery

2 Cloves Of Garlic

½ TSP Thyme Leaves

1 TSP Fajita Seasoning

50 Grams Mixed Peppers

25 Grams Cooked Pinto Beans (From Can, Rinsed)

25 Grams Frozen Soya Beans

25 Grams Frozen Peas

400 Mls Hot Water

1 Organic Vegetable Stock Cube

2 TBSP Tomato Puree

600 Grams Tomato Passata

Himalayan Pink Salt

Black Pepper

Peel and finely dice onion and carrot, wash celery and finely dice. Finely dice the peppers and measure out the rest of your ingredients.

In a small saucepan cook the penne pasta (according to pack instructions) and refresh in cold water to stop the pasta becoming overcooked.

Place a large stainless steel saucepan on a medium heat, add olive oil, onion, carrot, celery, garlic, thyme and fajita seasoning, sauté for 5 minutes, stirring to prevent colouring the vegetables.

Add the tomato puree, stir in and cook for a further minute before adding the hot water and stock cube. Bring to the boil and simmer for 10 minutes to ensure the more robust veggies are tender.

Add the peppers, soya beans, pinto beans, peas and passata. Heat through gently for 10 minutes, continually stirring, before finally adding the pre-cooked pasta. Season to taste with Himalayan pink salt and black pepper.

Adjust the consistency of this rustic soup with some hot water if required.

Soya beans are a good source of B vitamins and minerals, helping to support energy levels and stress-coping mechanism.

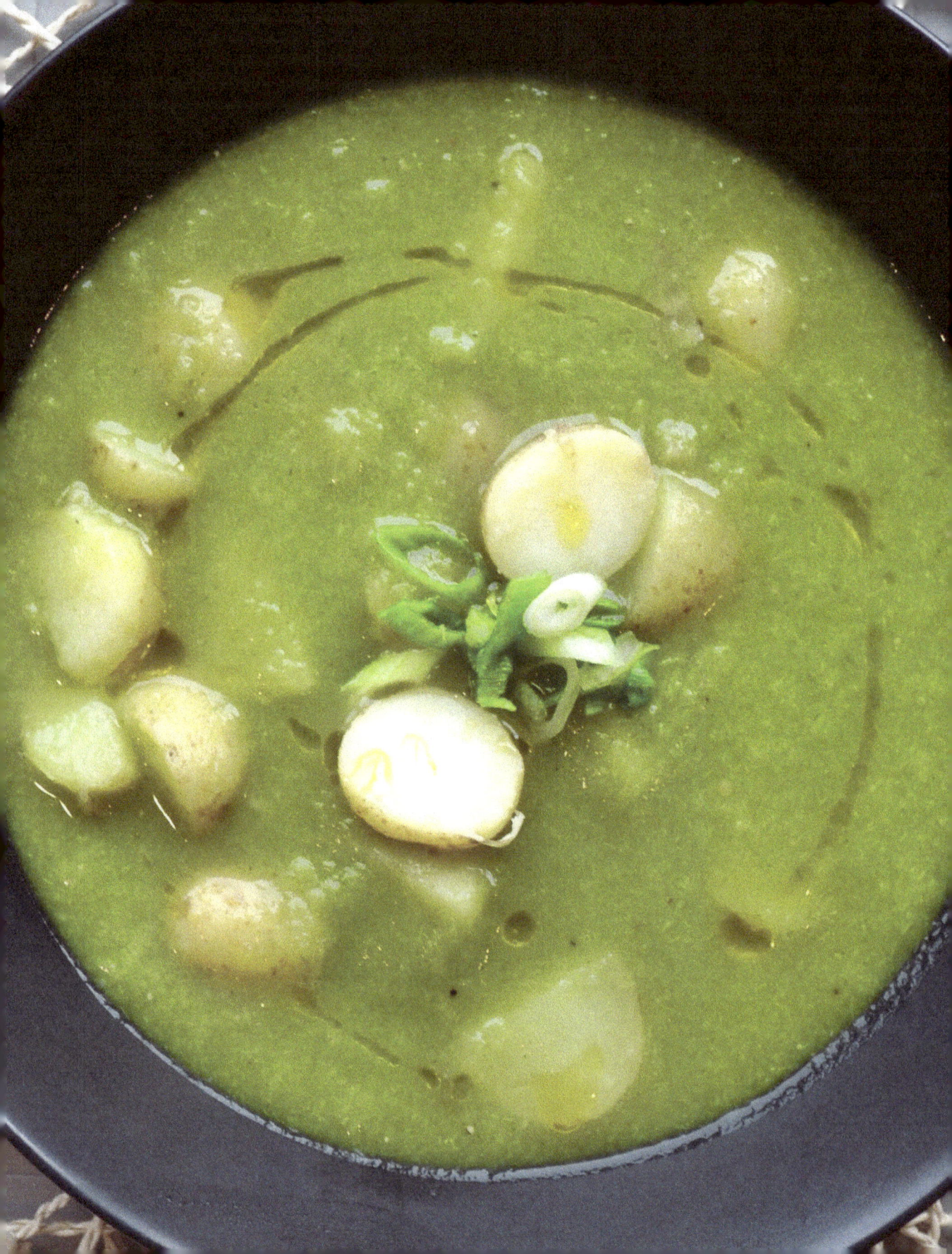

SIMPLE LEEK AND POTATO SOUP

SERVES 2

300 Grams Baby Potatoes

1 Leek

1 Organic Vegetable Stock Cube

1 Litre Hot Water

1 Spring Onion

Ground Himalayan Pink Salt

Freshly Ground Black Pepper

Wash the potatoes and place in a medium stainless steel saucepan and pour in the hot water. Put the pan on a high heat and boil the potatoes for 20 minutes or until they are just tender.

Remove the potatoes from the water with a slotted spoon and set aside.

Roughly chop and wash the leek and add to the potato water, along with the stock cube.

Bring the leeks to the boil and simmer for 10 minutes.

When the leeks are tender, blend with a handheld stick blender and season to taste with Himalayan pink salt and freshly ground black pepper.

Cut the baby potatoes into cubes and add to the pureed soup.

Finely slice the spring onion for garnish.

Potatoes contain tryptophan, an amino acid with natural sedative properties to calm the nervous system.

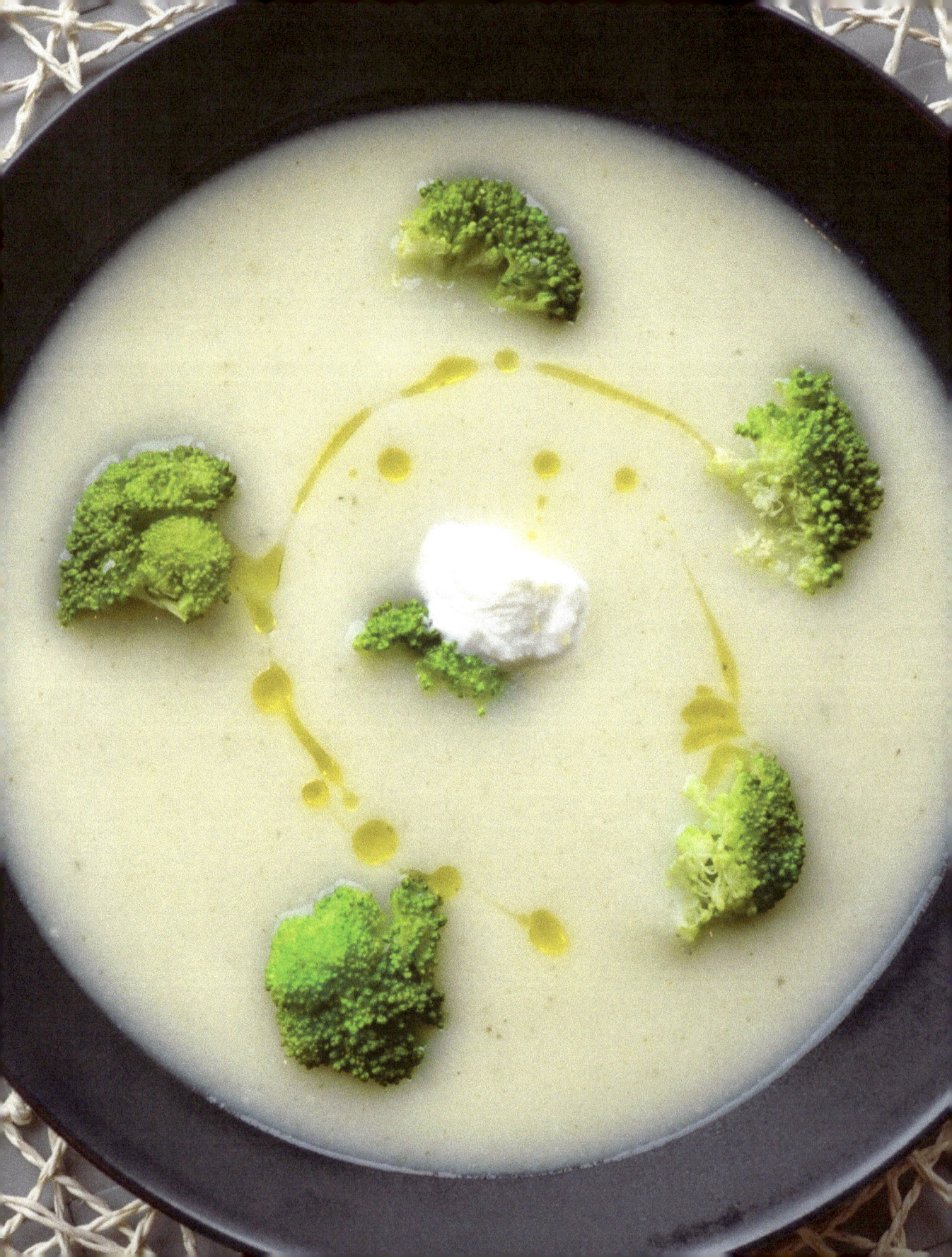

CAULIFLOWER AND BROCCOLI SOUP WITH SAGE AND GOATS CHEESE

SERVES 4

1 TBSP Extra Virgin Organic Olive Oil

1 Small Onion

1 Rib Of Celery

½ TSP Fresh Thyme Leaves

6 Sage Leaves

800 Grams Fresh Cauliflower Florets

200 Grams Fresh Small Broccoli Florets

60 Grams Goats Cheese (Preferably Organic and Made With Raw Goats Milk)

1 Organic Vegetable Stock Cube

1250 Mls Hot Water

Ground Himalayan Pink Salt

Freshly Ground Black Pepper

Peel and roughly chop onion, wash and roughly chop celery.

Finely chop the thyme and sage leaves.

Place a large stainless steel saucepan on a medium heat, add the olive oil, onion, celery, thyme and sage, sauté for 5 minutes to soften, then add the cauliflower, stock cube and hot water. Bring to the boil and simmer for 20 minutes or until all the vegetables are tender.

Blitz the soup with a handheld stick blender, season to taste with ground Himalayan pink salt and black pepper, add the goats cheese (saving a little for garnish) and give it another blitz until silky smooth and creamy.

In a small stainless steel saucepan blanch the broccoli florets in boiling water until tender, but still green and vibrant, drain the broccoli and add to the soup and serve.

Broccoli promotes collagen synthesis and strengthens immune system.

CARROT, LENTIL AND GINGER SOUP

SERVES 2

1 TBSP Extra Virgin Organic Olive Oil

1 Small Onion

2 Cloves Garlic

1 Thumb-size Piece Of Ginger

4 Medium Carrots

100 Grams Red Lentils

1 Organic Vegetable Stock Cube

1 Litre Of Hot Water

Ground Himalayan Pink Salt

Freshly Ground Black Pepper

Peel and roughly chop onion, garlic, carrots and ginger.

Place a medium stainless steel saucepan on a medium heat, add olive oil, onion, garlic, carrots and ginger, sauté for 5 minutes, stirring regularly.

Pour in hot water and add stock cube. Bring to the boil and simmer for 10 minutes or until the carrots are just tender, then add the lentils and simmer for a further 10 minutes.

Ensure lentils are soft before blitzing the soup with a handheld stick blender. Season to taste with freshly ground Himalayan pink salt and black pepper, and give it another blitz until silky smooth.

Adjust the consistency with a some hot water if necessary.

Lentils are an excellent food which help oxygenate the blood and aid in the release of cellular energy.

CHICKEN BONE BROTH

2 Organic Free Range Chicken Carcasses.

2 Onions

2 Carrots

2 Ribs of Celery

½ A Leek

1 Full Bulb Of Garlic

5 Bay Leaves

3 Large Sprigs Thyme

3 Large Sprigs Rosemary

2 TBSP Apple Cider Vinegar (With Mother Culture)

3 Litres Of Filtered Water

Roast the carcasses in the oven at 230 degrees Celsius for 15 minutes, then transfer to your slow cooker.

Wash and roughly chop all the veg (no need to peel anything) and add to the slow cooker with the remaining ingredients. Cook on the high setting for 24 to 48 hours (the longer the better).

Allow to cool slightly before straining the liquid into a jug or container that will fit in your fridge. After 2 hours of further cooling, put the broth into the fridge overnight. The next day, scrape off the fat and your broth is ready for use, as a drink or in soups.

Bone broth boosts detoxification and maintains healthy skin.

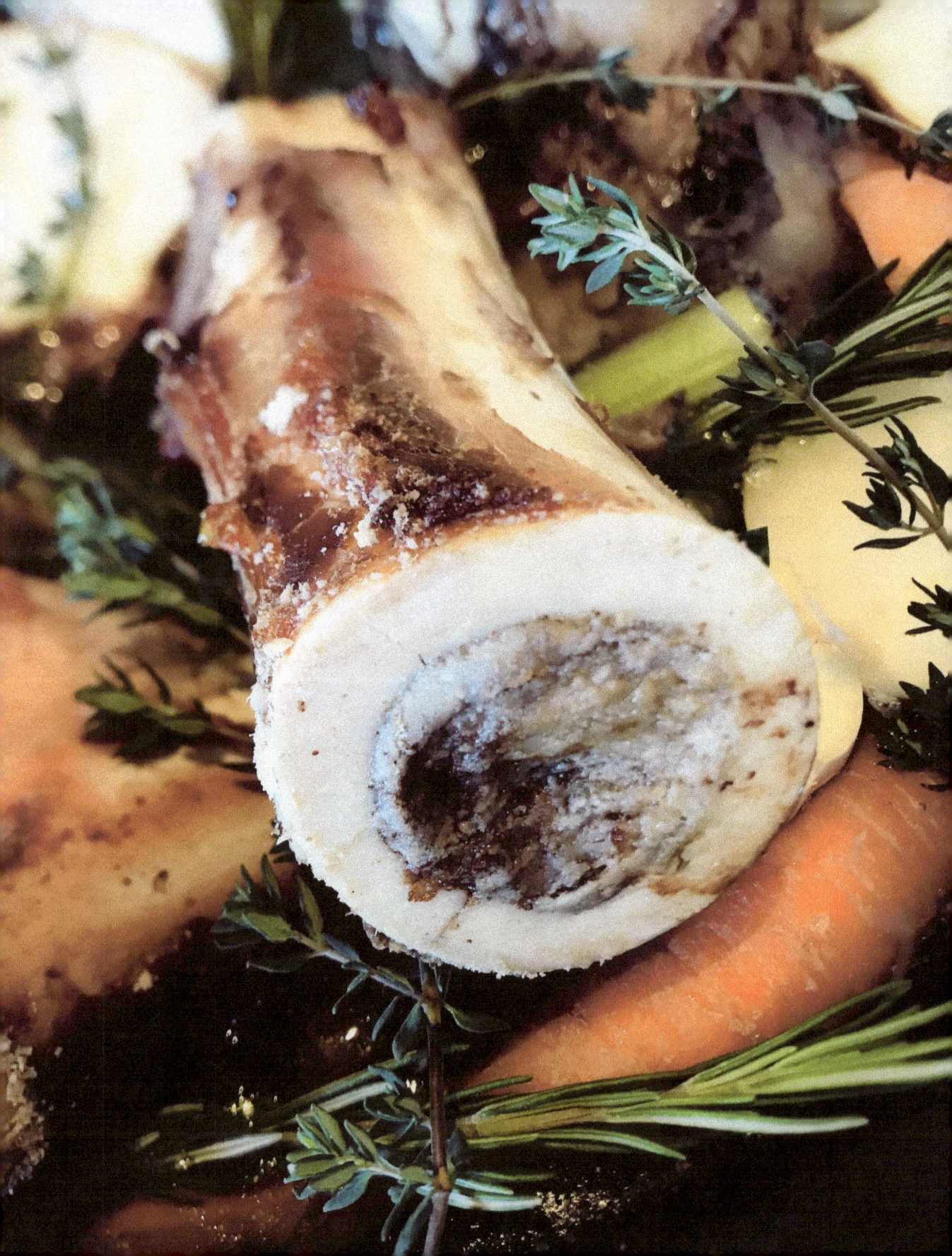

BEEF BONE BROTH

2 Grass-fed Organic Beef Shin Marrow Bones

2 Onions

2 Carrots

2 Ribs of Celery

½ A Leek

1 Full Bulb Of Garlic

5 Bay Leaves

3 Large Sprigs Thyme

3 Large Sprigs Rosemary

2 TBSP Apple Cider Vinegar (With Mother Culture)

3 Litres Of Filtered Water

Roast the bones in the oven at 230 degrees Celsius for 15 minutes, then transfer to your slow cooker.

Wash and roughly chop all the veg (no need to peel anything) and add to the slow cooker with the remaining ingredients. Cook on the high setting for 24 to 48 hours (the longer the better).

Allow to cool slightly before straining the liquid into a jug or container that will fit in your fridge. After 2 hours of further cooling, put the broth into the fridge overnight. The next day, scrape off the fat and your broth is ready for use, as a drink or in soups.

Bone broth supports gut health and protects joints thanks to its natural source of collagen.

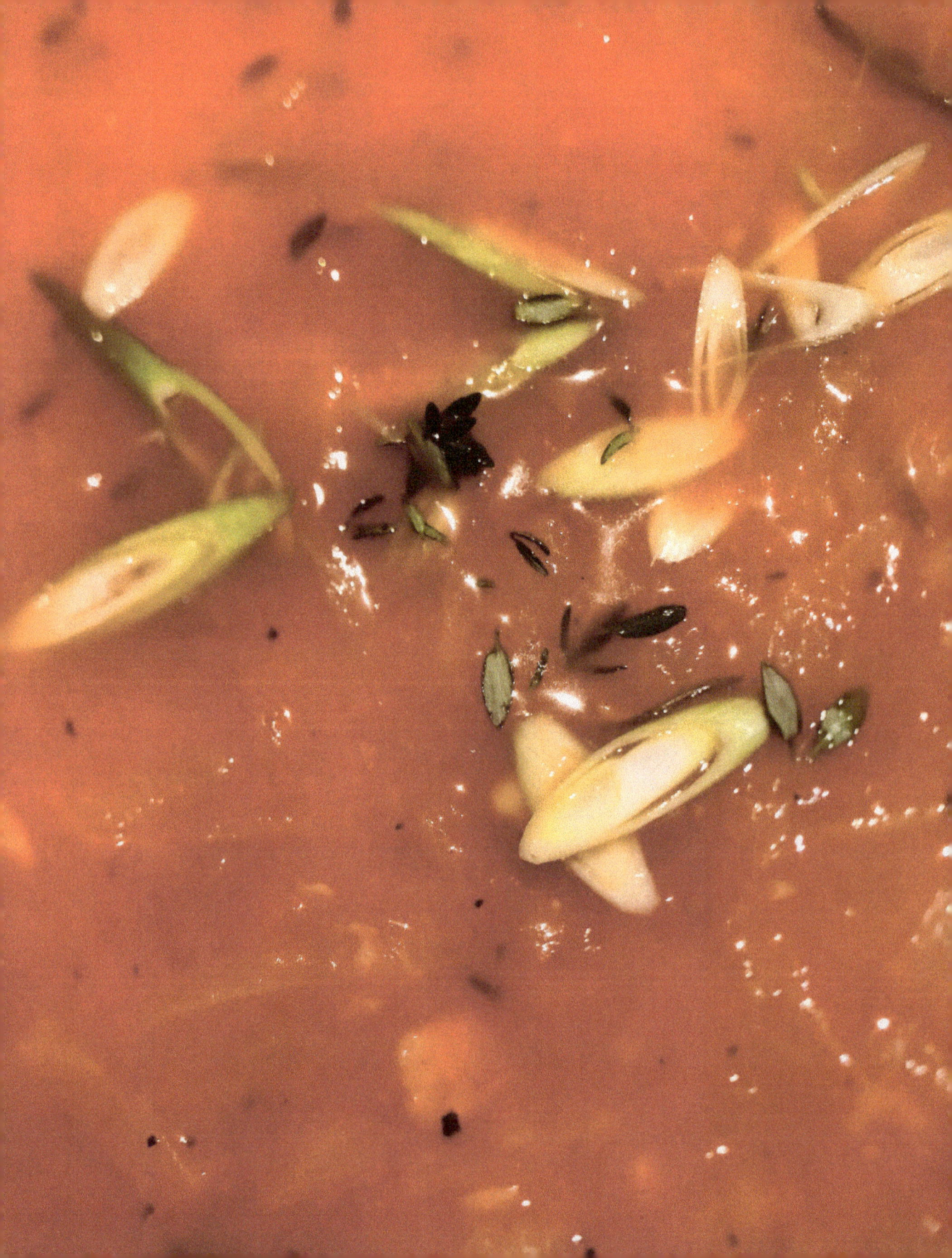

FRENCH ONION SOUP

SERVES 4

3 Large Onions

2 Litres of Boiling Water

1 Large Sprig Of Rosemary

1 Large Sprig Of Thyme

3 Bay Leaves

4 Cloves of Crushed Garlic

70 Grams of Tomato Puree

1 Litre of Beef Bone Broth (SEE PAGE 105) *or*
2 Organic Beef Stock Cubes and 1 Litre Of
Water

Ground Himalayan Pink Salt

Freshly Ground Black Pepper

1 Spring Onion Sliced

Peel and finely slice the onions and place in a medium size saucepan with the boiling water, rosemary, thyme, bay leaves, and garlic, bring to the boil and then simmer for 90 minutes. The liquid should have reduced by half.

Add the tomato puree and the bone broth or stock & water, stir well and simmer for a further 60 minutes.

Season to taste with the Himalayan salt and black pepper, adjust consistency with some hot water if necessary & Garnish with sliced spring onion.

Onions are a great pre-biotic food, which feed the good gut bacteria.

OUR
DAILY
BREAD

When it comes to real bread, we need to get back to basics! When I read the ingredients on a loaf of bread from the supermarket, it really frustrates me. All these E numbers and additives are put in to achieve the light, soft and fluffy texture, most people associate with high quality. The modern wheat, used in most store-bought bread nowadays has been modified and hybridised over the years, resulting in a much higher gluten content, which may be compromising gut health in many people. Organic spelt is the ancient grain that has been used for thousands of years, untouched by modern processing methods, and it is this grain that I have chosen to offer a small selection of homemade bread recipes that you can easily include in your everyday meals.

Please note that spelt does contain gluten and is not suitable for anyone who is gluten intolerant or celiac.

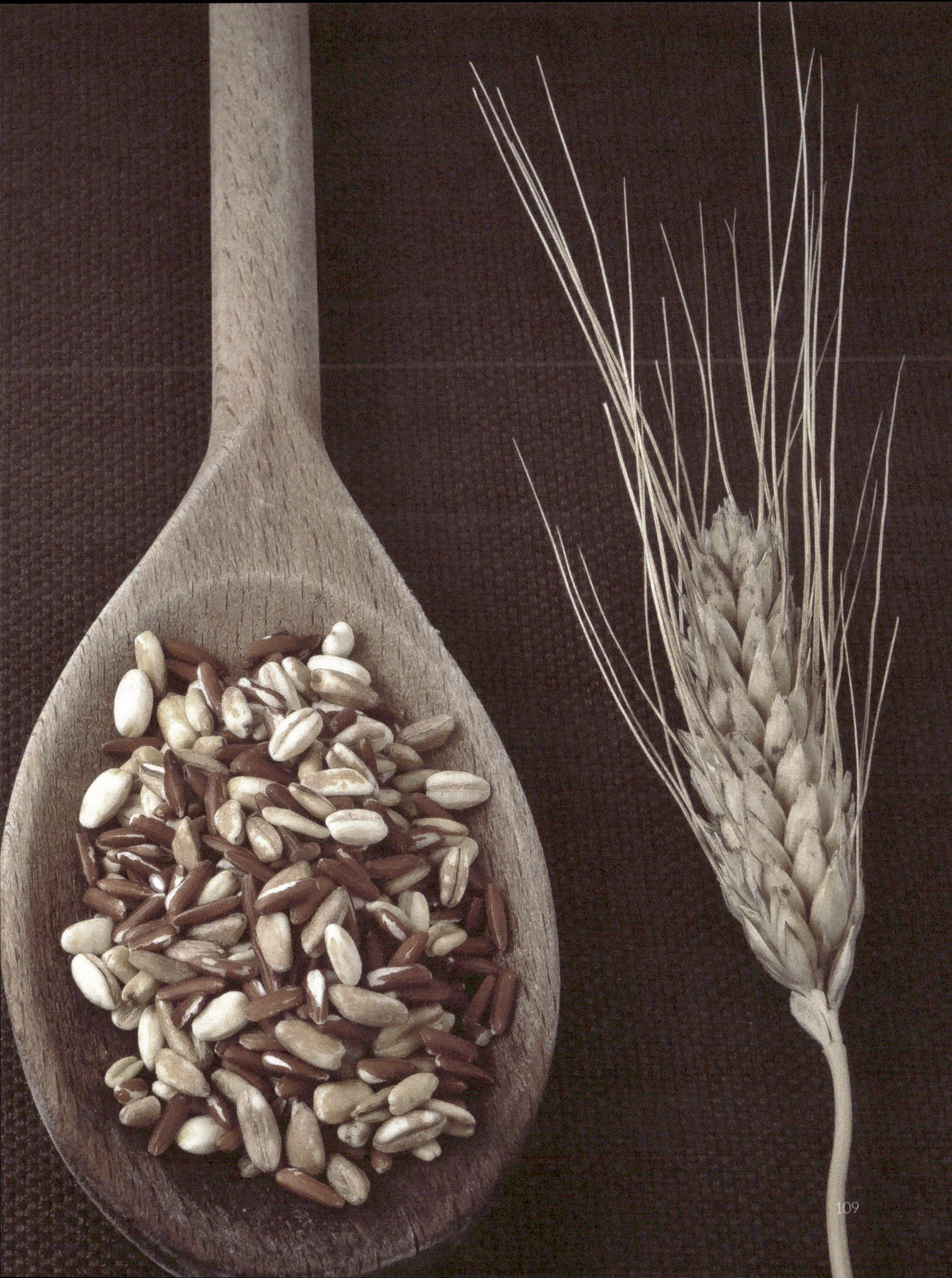

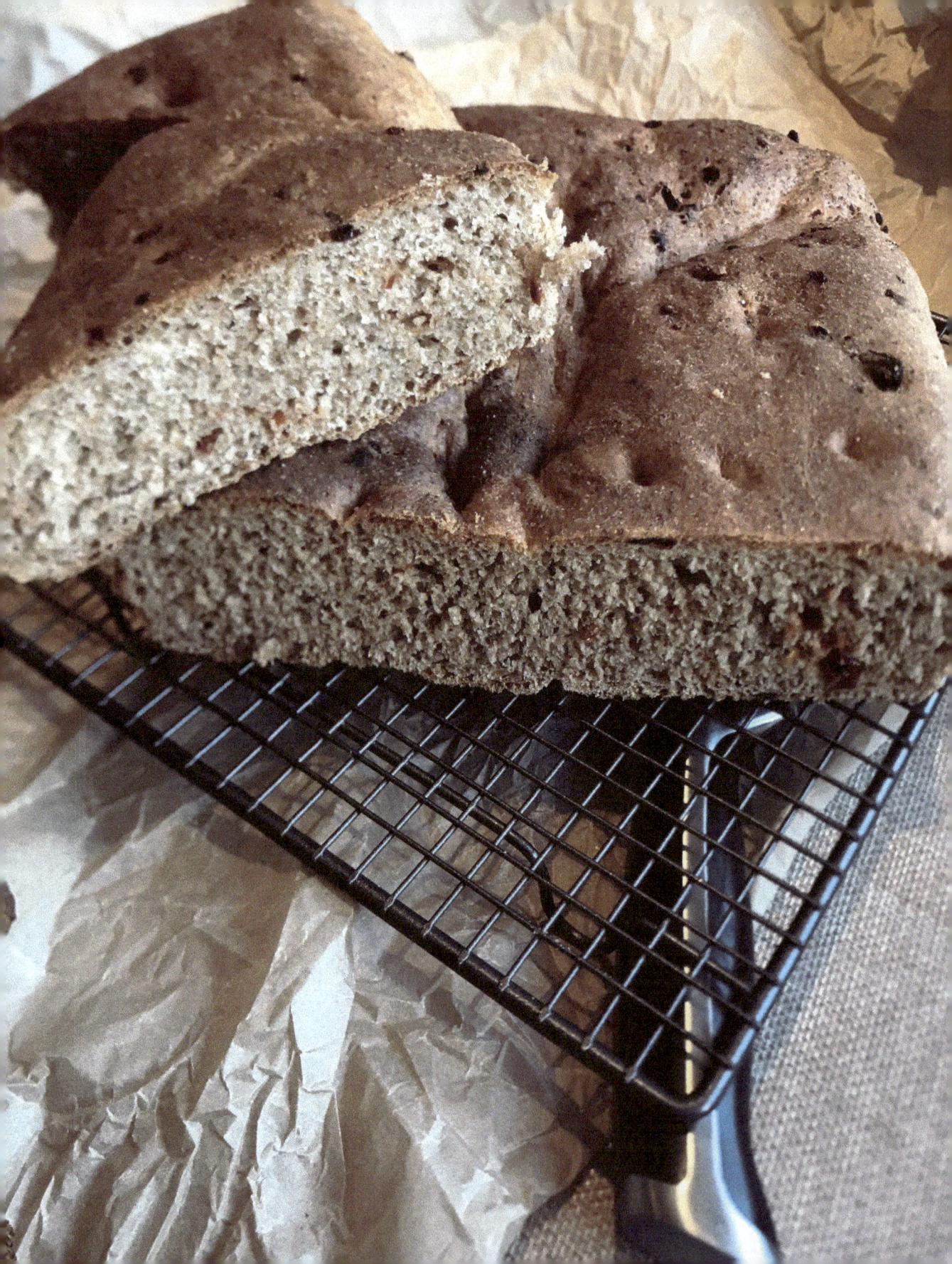

SUN-DRIED TOMATO FOCACCIA BREAD

500 grams organic wholemeal spelt flour

14 grams fast acting dried yeast

1 tsp ground Himalayan pink salt

350 mls lukewarm water

3 tbsp organic extra virgin olive oil + more for greasing and brushing on top

4 sun-dried Tomatoes (dry, not in oil)

Start by rehydrating the sun-dried tomatoes in boiling water for at least 15 mins.

Grease (with olive oil) and lightly flour a 320 mm × 220 mm non-stick traybake tray, ensuring all surfaces are covered including the sides, and shake off any excess flour.

Put the spelt flour, yeast and salt into a food mixer with the dough hook attachment and turn on to the lowest speed for 1 minute.

Stop the mixer and add the water and olive oil. Using a spatula mix manually to bring all the ingredients together. Now turn on the mixer to the lowest setting again and let the machine do the kneading for 10 minutes.

Whilst the dough is kneading you can drain the tomatoes, and chop them as fine as possible.

Spelt provides slow release energy.

After 10 minutes of kneading, add the sun-dried tomatoes to the dough and allow to mix for a further minute.

Lightly flour a clean surface and your hands too, remove the dough from the mixer and knead for 1 further minute by hand, this ensures an even distribution of the fine tomatoes. (If the dough gets a little sticky just sprinkle over some more flour.)

Now transfer the dough into your prepared tray, pressing with your fingertips, ensuring the dough reaches all sides of the tray, and it is an even depth all over.

Cover with a clean tea towel and allow to prove in a warm place e.g. top of the hob, for 45 minutes. Meanwhile preheat the oven to 220 °C.

After proving, the dough should have almost doubled in size. Brush with a little olive oil and put into the oven. Bake for 10 minutes at 220 °C and then turn the temperature down to 190 °C, and bake for a further 20 minutes.

Remove bread from the tray and allow to rest on a wire rack for at least 15 minutes before cutting.

Enjoy!

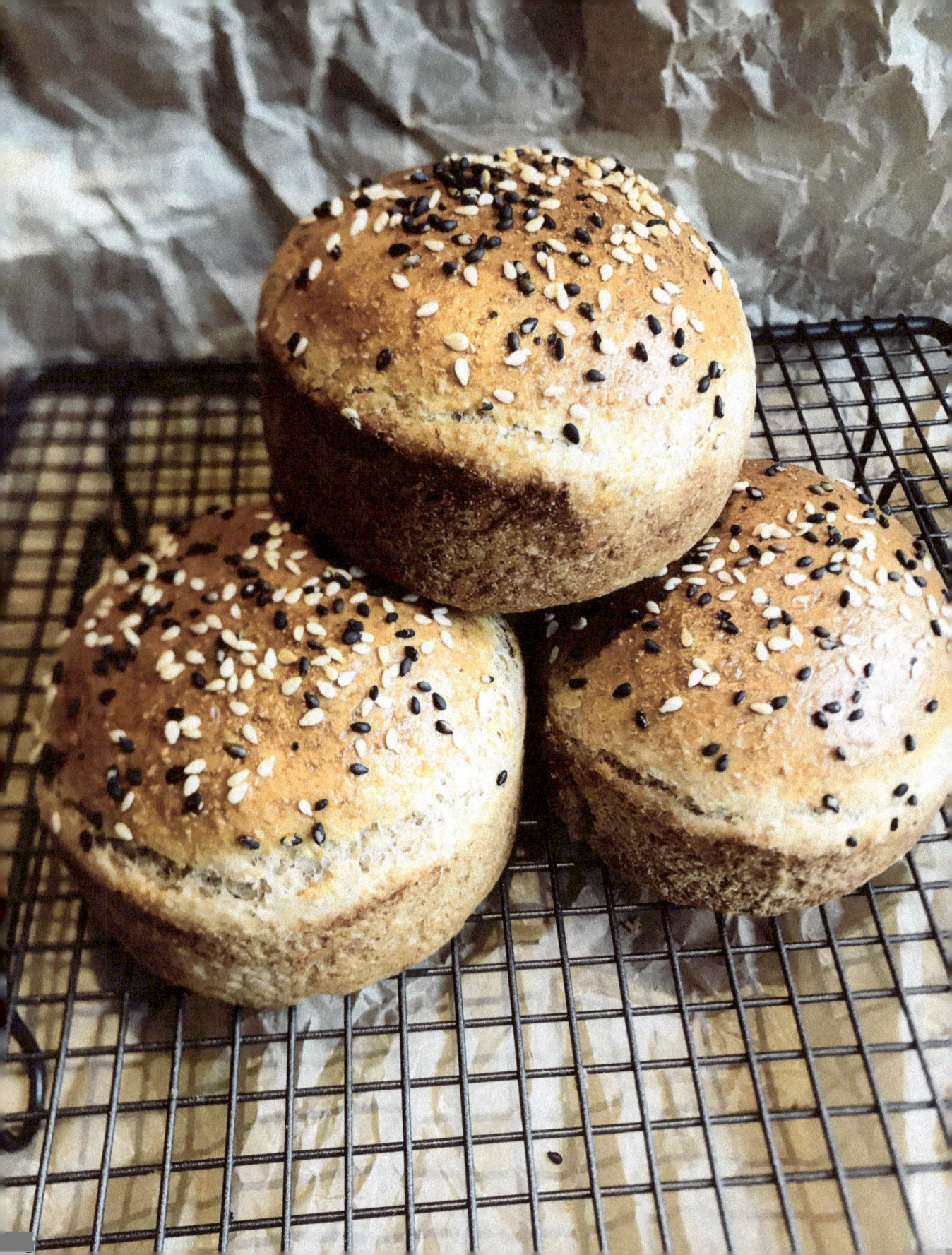

SPELT BURGER BUNS

250 grams organic wholemeal spelt flour

7 grams fast acting dried yeast

½ tsp ground Himalayan pink salt

160 mls lukewarm water

2 tbsp organic extra virgin olive oil

1 tbsp raw organic honey

1 organic egg yolk + a splash of water (eggwash)

Black and white sesame seeds

Put the spelt flour, yeast and salt into a food mixer with the dough hook attachment and turn on to the lowest speed for 1 minute.

Stop the mixer and add the water, olive oil & honey. Using a spatula mix manually to bring all the ingredients together. Now turn on the mixer to the lowest setting again and let the machine do the kneading for 10 minutes, stop the mixer, remove dough hook, allow the dough to prove for 1 hour in a warm place, covered with a tea towel.

After the first prove, remove from bowl,

Lightly flour a clean surface and your hands too, remove the dough from the bowl and knead for 1 further minute by hand.

Cut the dough into 4 even size pieces, roll each one into a ball, using a little extra flour if required, and place each one into a greased (olive oil) 9 cm (diameter) stainless steel cooking ring, sitting on a baking sheet lined with a non-stick silicone mat. Allow to prove for a second time for 30 minutes in a warm place.

Preheat your oven to 200 °C. Mix your eggwash together with a pastry brush.

After the second prove, brush each bun with the eggwash and sprinkle on some black and white sesame seeds.

Bake in the oven for 18–20 minutes at 200 °C.

Remove from oven and allow to rest for at least 15 minutes on a wire rack.

Enjoy!

Wholegrain Spelt is a good source of nutrients, in particular B vitamins.

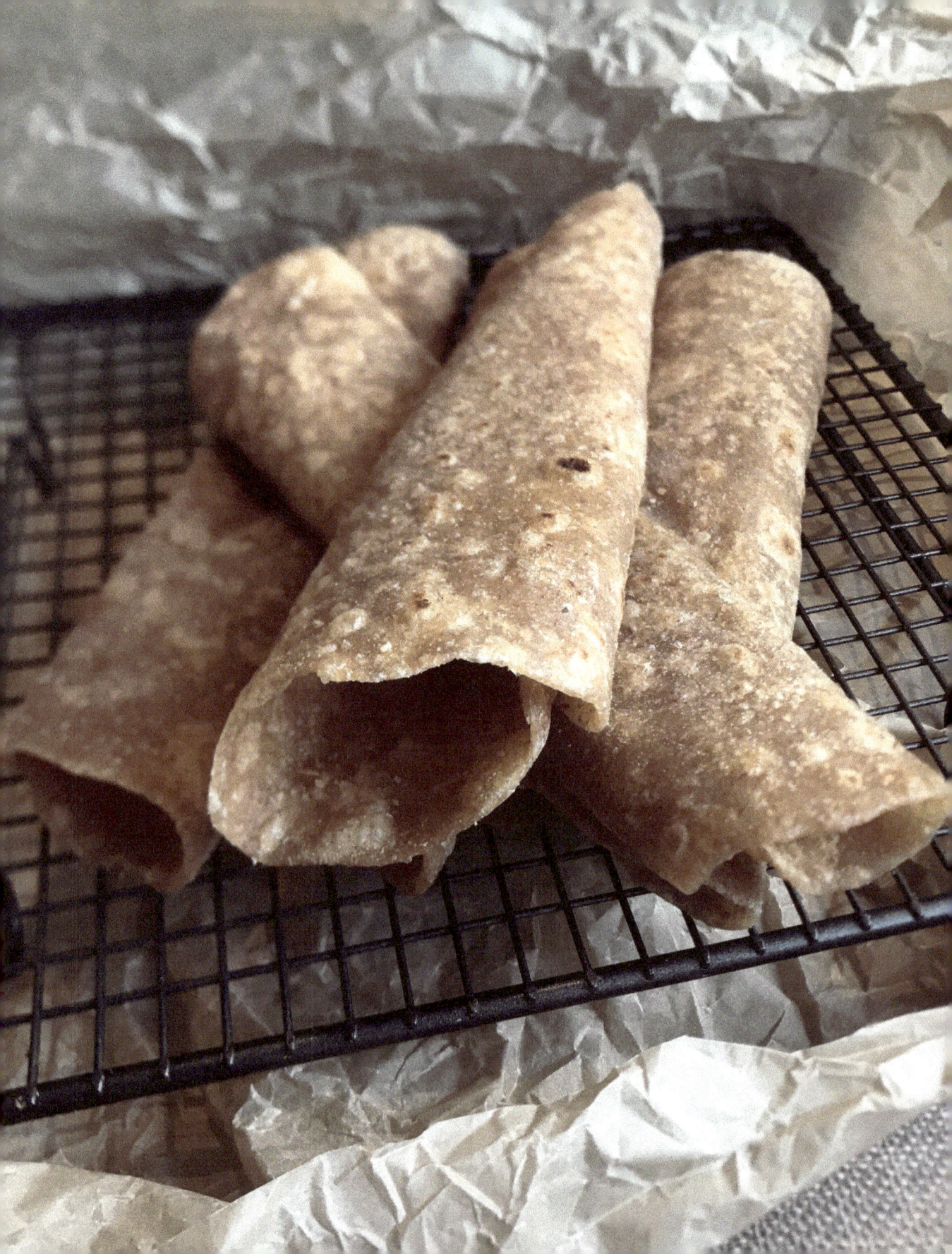

TORTILLA WRAP

MAKES 10 WRAPS

250 grams organic wholemeal spelt flour

4 tbsp extra virgin organic olive oil + more for cooking

½ tsp ground Himalayan pink salt

150 mls lukewarm water

In a large mixing bowl, mix all the ingredients together with clean hands, and knead for 2 minutes to a soft dough.

Wrap in cling film and allow to rest for 30 minutes.

Cut the dough into 10 equal size pieces and roll into balls with the aid of a little extra flour if necessary.

With a floured rolling pin and surface, roll each ball out to a very thin circular wrap and place under a tea towel to prevent drying out.

In a non-stick frying pan on a high heat, cook each wrap with a little olive oil for about 30 seconds each side. Placing each cooked wrap under the tea towel again to stop drying out.

Spelt is a healthy source of protein.

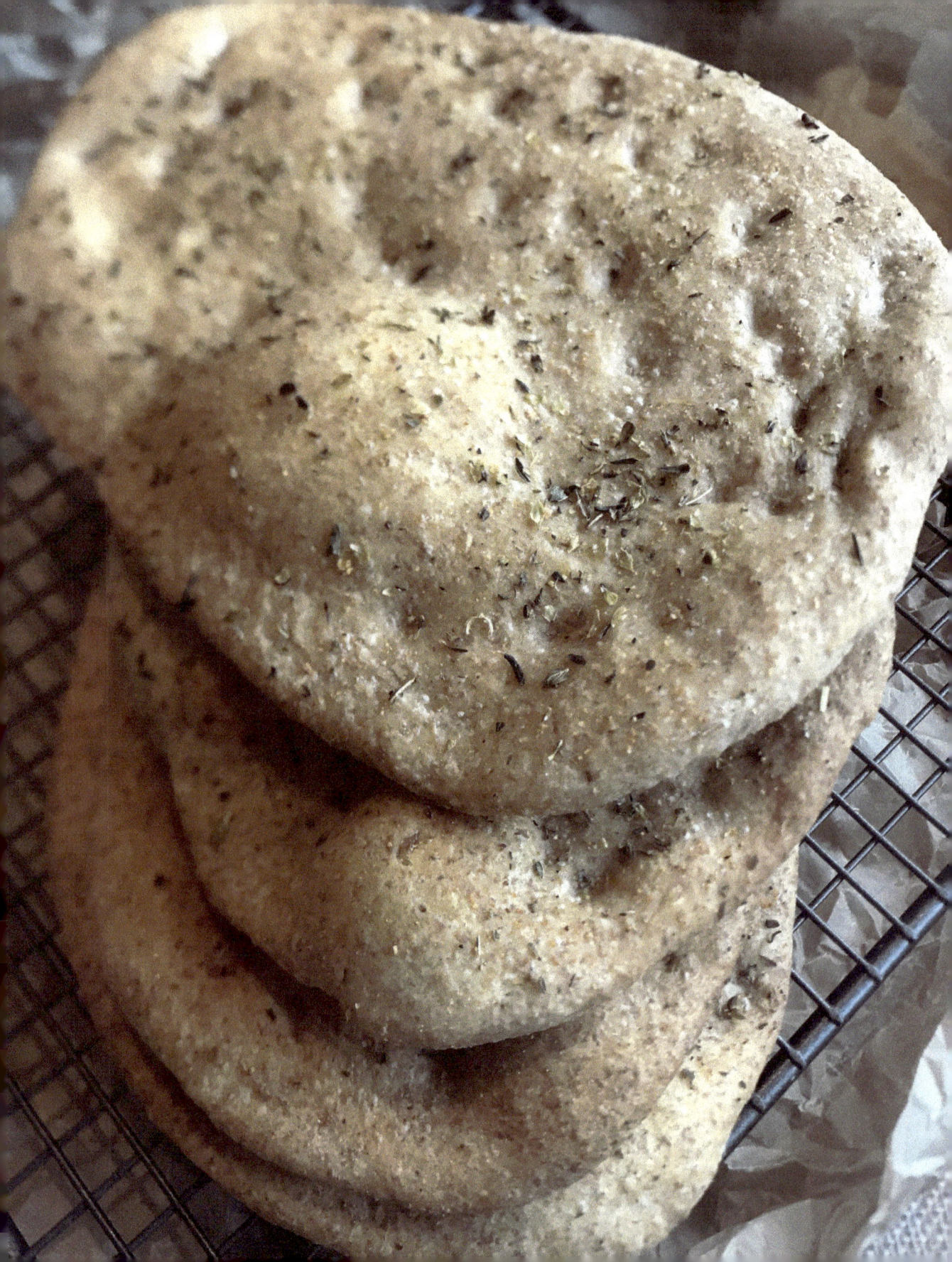

FLATBREAD

MAKES 8 FLATBREADS

280 grams organic wholegrain spelt flour

7 grams fast acting yeast

1 tsp baking powder

½ tsp ground Himalayan pink salt

4 tbsp extra virgin organic olive oil + more for cooking

175 mls lukewarm water

Garlic granules

Dried oregano

Put the flour, yeast, baking powder and salt in the food mixer (with the dough hook attachment) and mix on the slowest speed for 1 minute. Add the oil and water and manually mix with a spatula to bring the ingredients together, and then allow the machine to knead the dough, on the slowest speed for 10 minutes.

Remove the dough from the machine, shape into a ball manually and place in a lightly oiled (olive oil) bowl and cover with a clean tea towel, allow to prove in a warm place for 45 minutes.

After the first prove, lightly flour a clean surface and knock the gas out of the dough, roll into a log and cut into 8 equal sized pieces, manually roll into doughballs. With a floured rolling pin, roll each ball into an oval flatbread about 5 mm thick. Prod each one with your fingers to create little divots, now brush with olive oil and from a height, very lightly season with garlic granules and dried oregano, allow to stand for a further 30 minutes.

Preheat your oven to 200 °C , Lightly brush a silicone baking sheet with olive oil and place 2 or 3 flatbreads on it, or as many as you can fit comfortably, bake for 8–9 minutes, repeat process until all your flatbreads are baked.

Spelt contains less gluten than conventional wheat. It is highly water soluble and easier to digest.

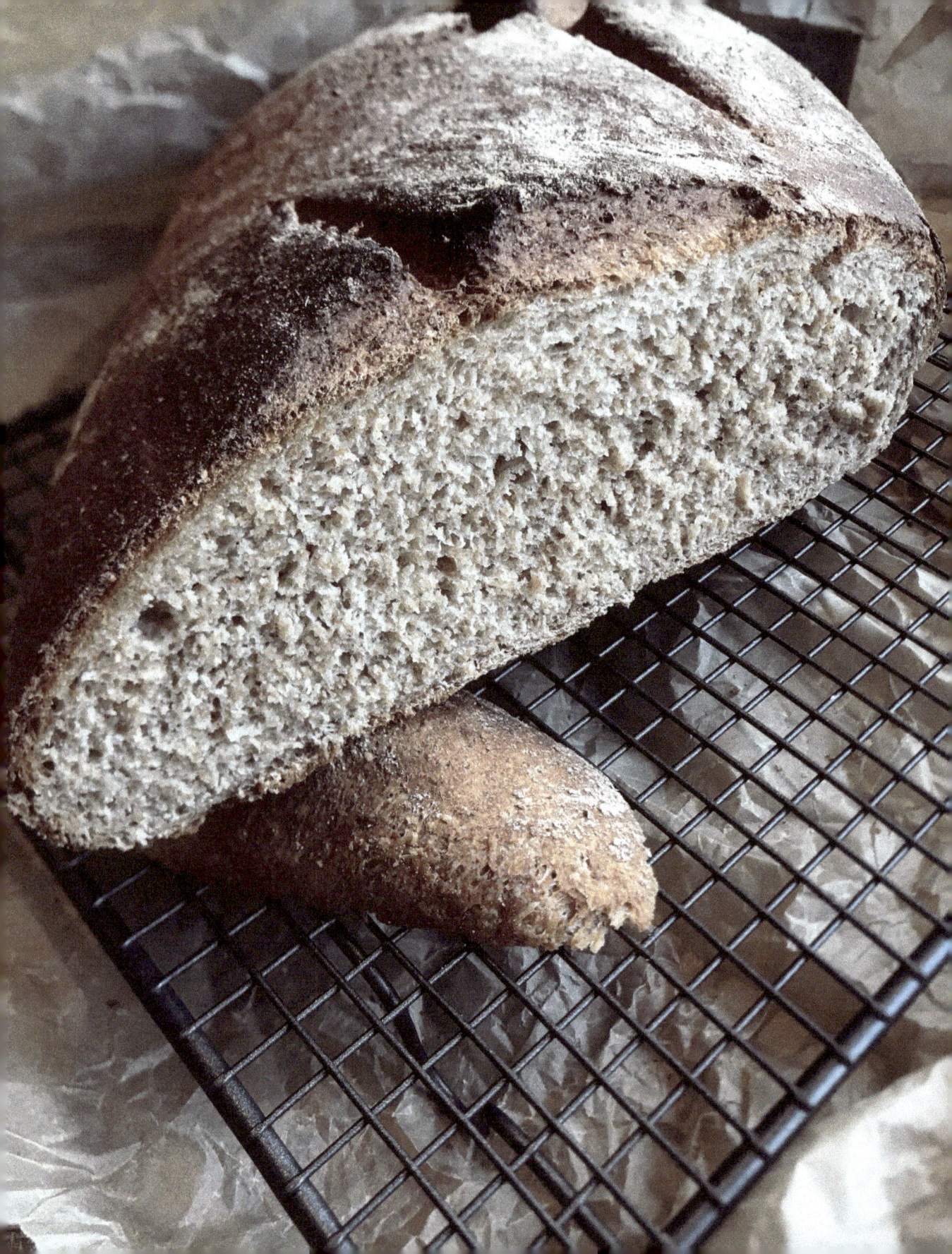

SPELT LOAF

500 grams organic wholemeal spelt flour

1tbsp ground Himalayan pink salt

14 grams fast acting yeast

1 tbsp raw organic honey

350 mls lukewarm water

Put the flour, salt and yeast into the food mixer with the dough hook attachment, mix at the slowest speed for 1 minute, stop and add the honey and water and manually bring the ingredients together with a spatula, before restarting the mixer on the slowest speed for a 10 minute knead.

Remove the dough from the bowl, and knead by hand on a floured surface, roll into a ball and place back in the mixer bowel, cover with a tea towel and leave to prove for 1 hour in a warm place.

Turn the dough out onto a floured surface, press and fold into a log shape, place onto an oiled and lighlty floured silicone baking sheet, sitting on the oven tray you plan to use, pinch the ends of the loaf and cover with a tea towel for its second prove of 30 minutes.

Preheat your oven to 230 °C. After the loaf has proven, take a serrated bread knife and make two cross cuts on top of the loaf and place in the hot oven and bake for 15 minutes at 230 °C, then turn the temperature to 200 for a further 15 minutes. Remove from the oven and rest on a wire rack for at least 20 minutes before cutting.

Wholegrain spelt helps balance blood sugar levels.

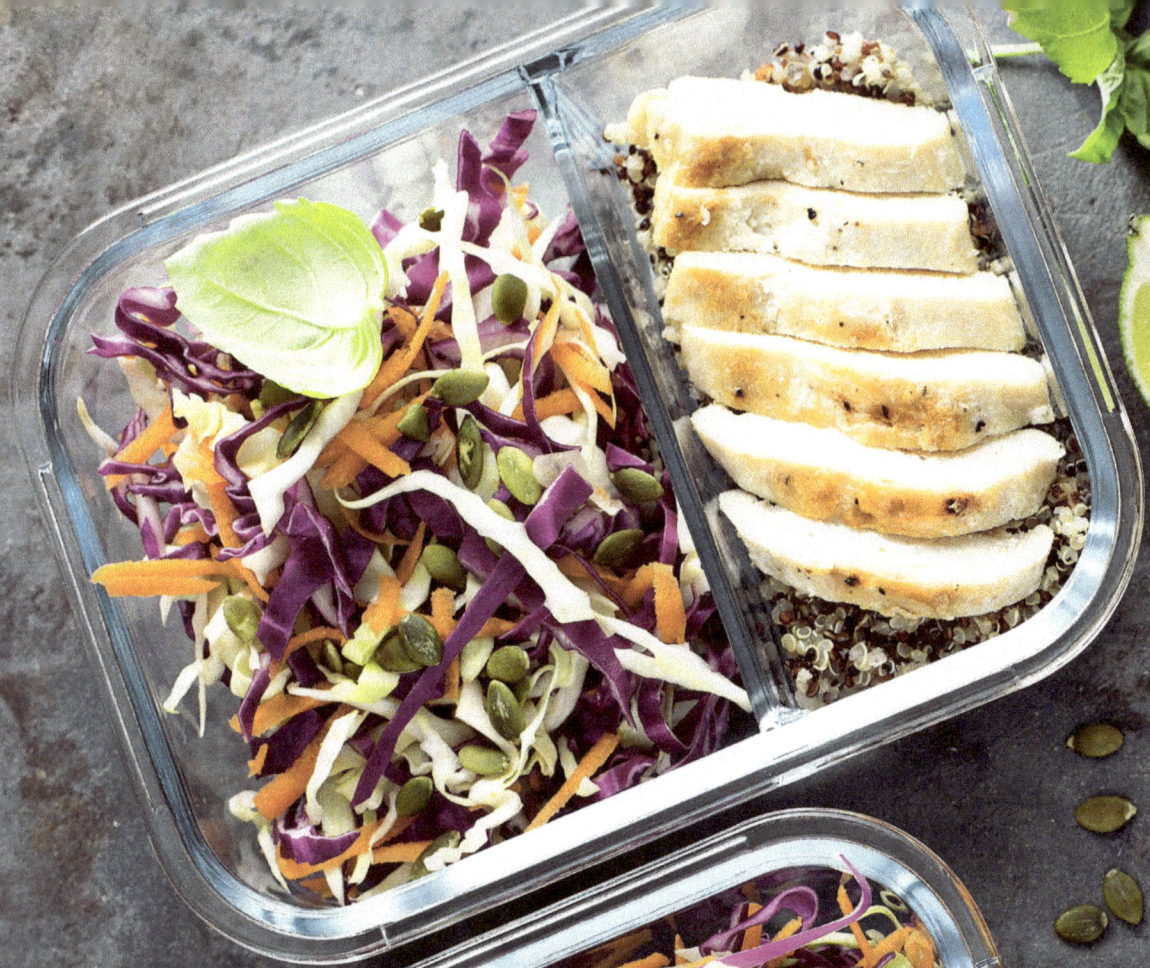

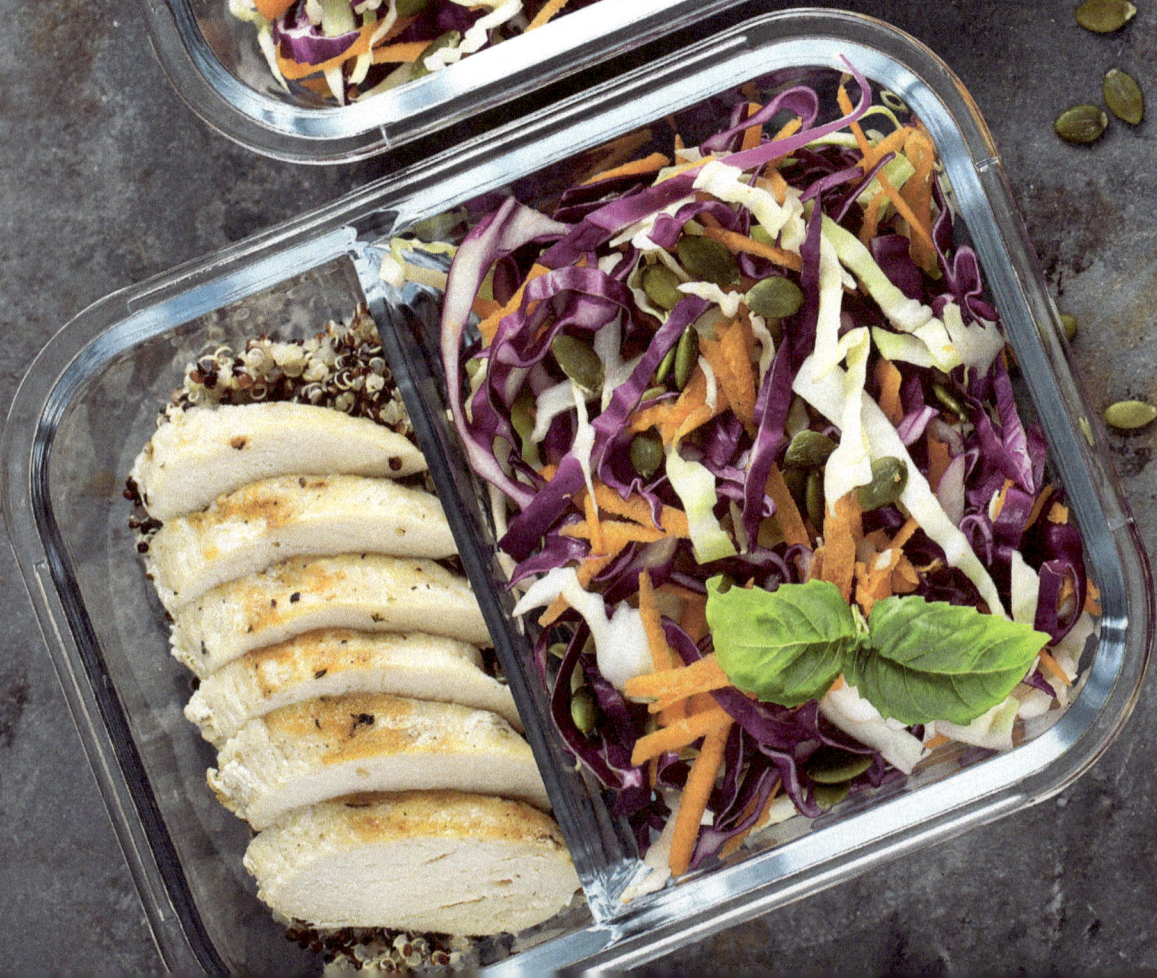

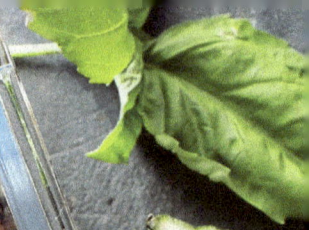

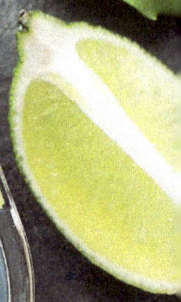

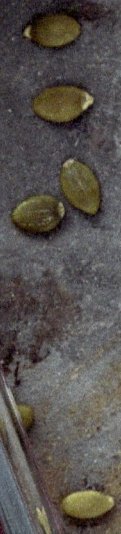

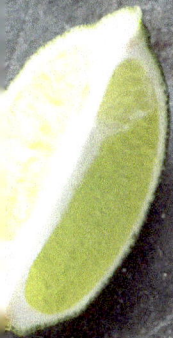

LUSH LUNCHES

Lunchtime is when many people make bad food choices, mainly down to convenience. I hope these ideas will inspire you, not only to try the recipes, but also create your own healthy dishes, prepared in advance, to combat the temptation of fast food.

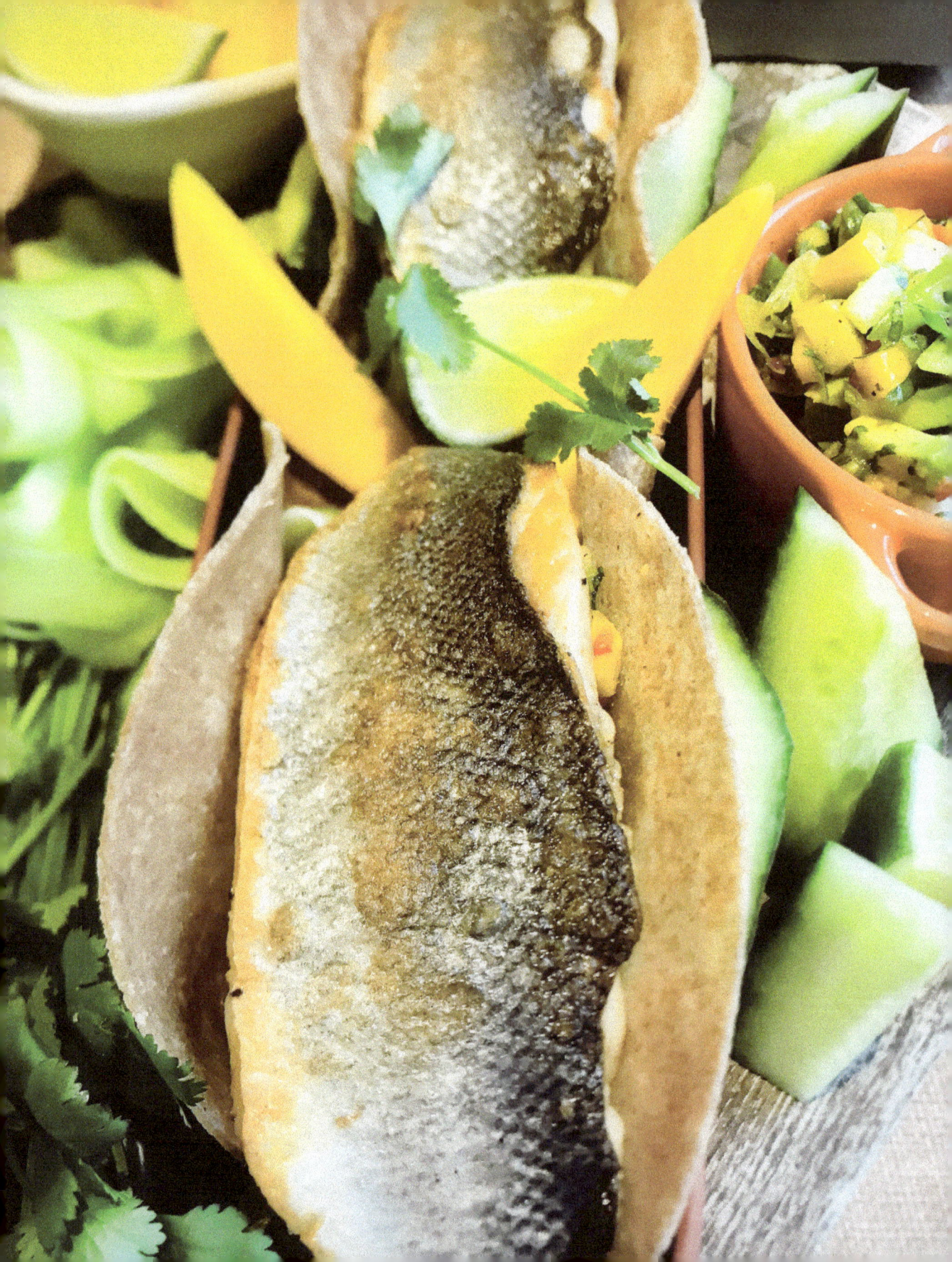

CARIBBEAN SEABASS TACOS WITH MANGO & CHILLI SALSA

SERVES 1–2

2 fresh seabass fillets (descaled and deboned)

¼ fresh pineapple

1 ripe fresh mango

1 medium sized red chilli

2 spring onions

20 grams fresh coriander

2 cloves garlic

2 limes (juice & zest)

1 avocado

2 tbsp extra virgin organic olive oil + more for cooking

1 cucumber

Ground Himalayan pink salt

Freshly ground black pepper

2 spelt tortillas (SEE PAGE 115)

FOR THE SALSA

Peel & finely dice pineapple, peel & remove stone of mango and finely dice, deseed and very finely dice the chilli, wash and finely slice the spring onions, finely chop the coriander (including the stocks), peel and chop the garlic with a pinch of salt to form a paste, peel and dice half the avocado, zest 1 lime and extract the juice. Place all ingredients in a mixing bowl, add the olive oil and season with black pepper and a little salt (remembering that salt was added to the garlic) and mix thoroughly, check the seasoning by tasting and adjust to your liking.

Mash the other half of the avocado with a small squeeze of lime. Top and tail the cucumber, and make ribbons with a speed peeler, and dress with another squeeze of lime.

Make perfect circular tacos by using a saucer as a stencil to cut around the spelt tortilla with a knife.

Place a large non-stick frying pan on a high heat. Rub your seabass fillets with a little olive oil and season with salt and pepper, when the pan is very hot, place the fillets skin side down and press lightly with your fingertips, cook on high for 2–3 minutes before turning and cooking for another 2 minutes and then remove pan from heat.

Fill your soft spelt tacos with layers of mashed avocado, cucumber ribbons, salsa and finally your beautiful seabass fillets.

Seabass is a semi-oily fish, It has a good balance of the anti-inflammatory omega-3 fats and high quality protein, as well as a plethora of vitamins and minerals.

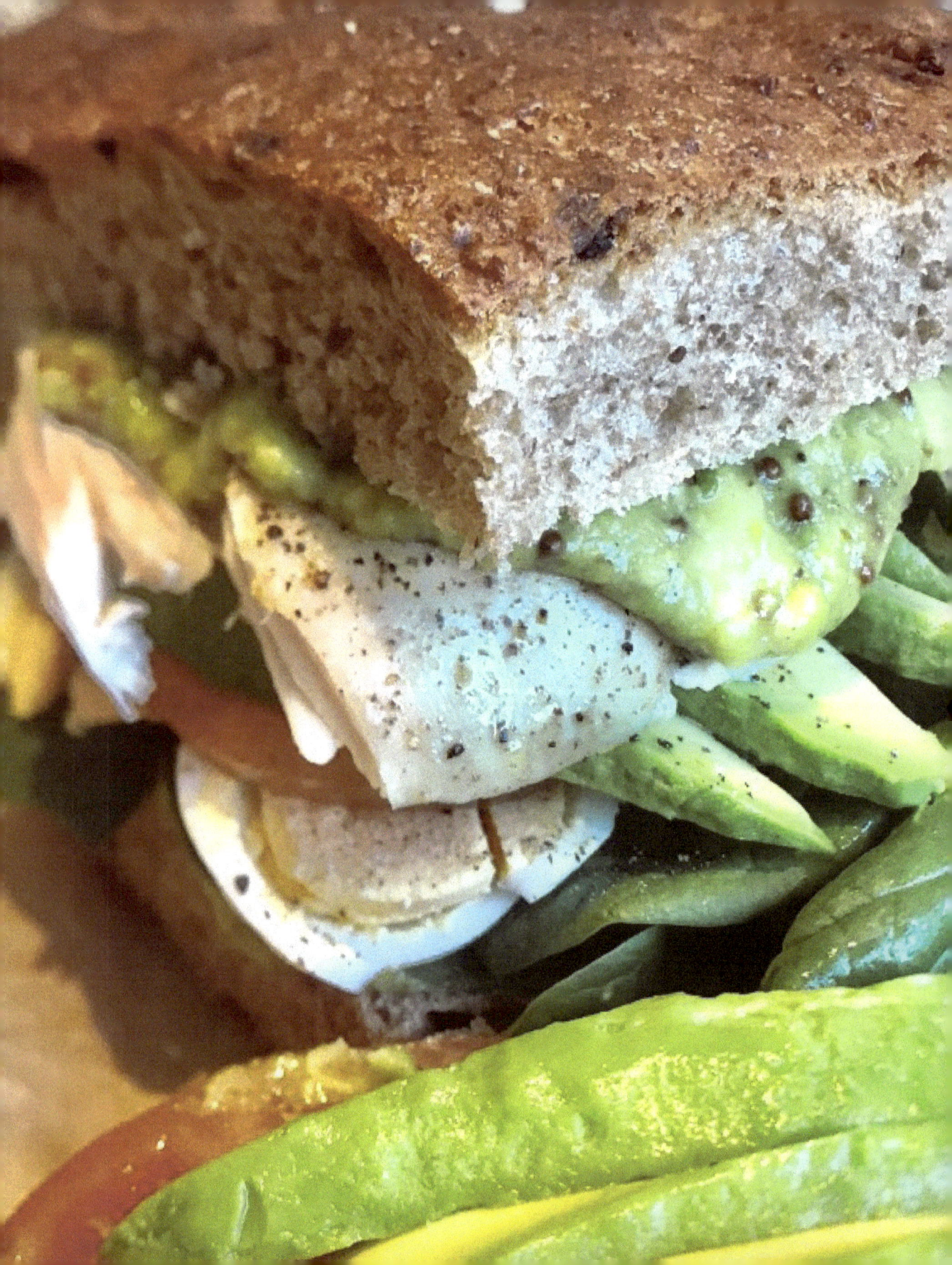

CALIFORNIAN CLUB SANDWICH

SERVES 1

FOR THE AVIOLI

½ avocado

1 tsp wholegrain mustard

1 tbsp raw organic honey

1 tbsp lemon juice

Ground Himalayan salt, and freshly ground black pepper

1 square of sun dried tomato focaccia (spelt) bread – (SEE PAGE 111)

1 hard-boiled egg, peeled and sliced

1 thick slice of beef tomato

Small handful of baby spinach

½ sliced avocado

100 grams of roast organic chicken breast (hot)

Ground Himalayan salt, and freshly ground black pepper

Parchment paper

Put the avocado in a pestle & mortar, bash and mix until pureed, add the honey, mustard, lemon juice & mix well, season to taste.

Cut your focaccia square in half and spread each side with the Avioli.

Starting with the spinach, begin layering up the sandwich, seasoning each layer as you go, followed by the sliced avocado, egg, tomato and chicken. Put the top on and wrap the club in parchment paper and place in a hot oven for 5 minutes, to warm and soften the focaccia bread.

Dig in with a knife and fork {:

Chicken contains all the B vitamins which help the body produce energy.

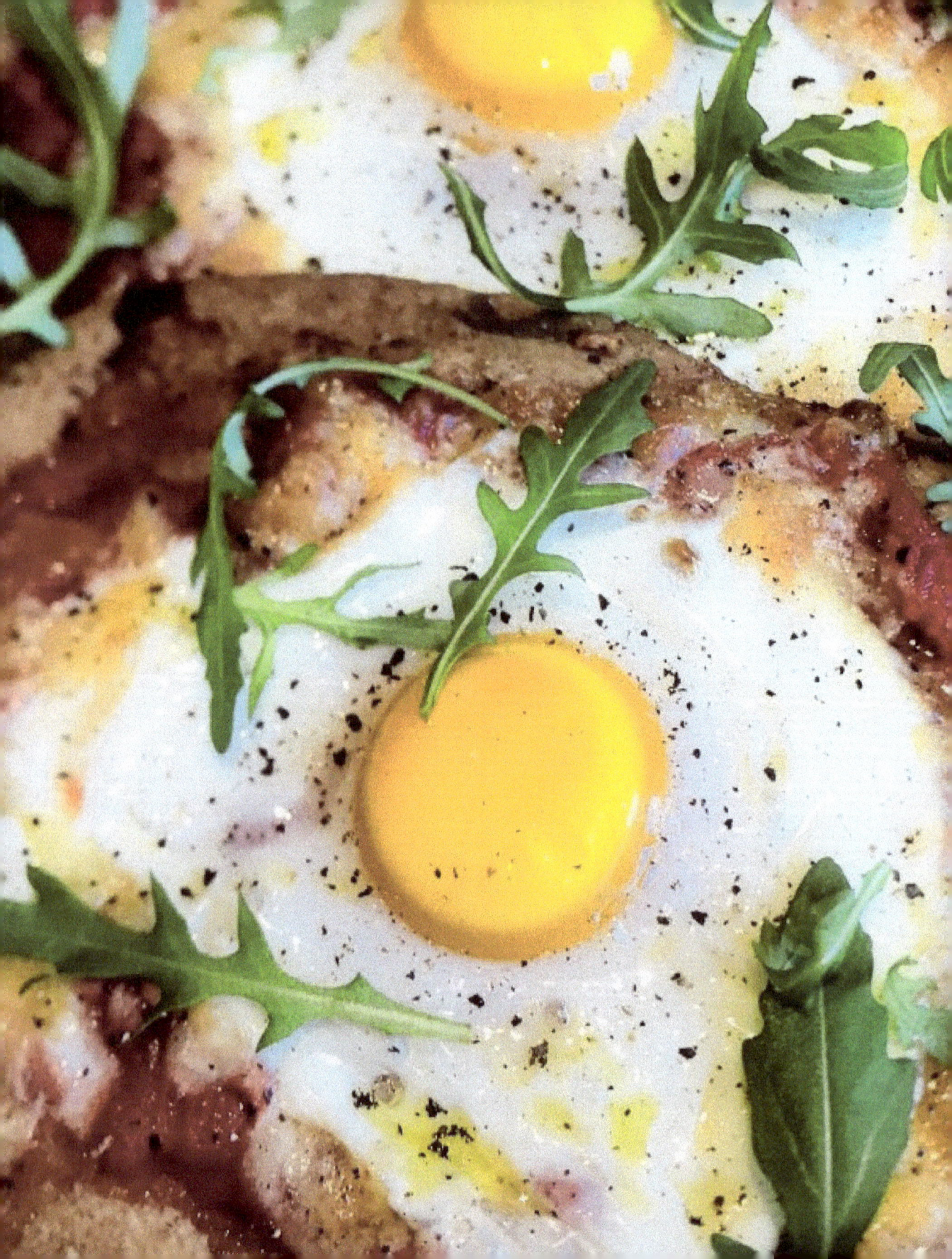

EGGY FLATBREAD PIZZA

SERVES 2

2 *spelt flatbreads* (SEE PAGE 117)

Organic pizza sauce

Organic cheddar

2 organic eggs

Rocket

Organic extra virgin Olive oil

Ground Himalayan pink salt

Freshly ground black pepper

Preheat your oven to 200 °C.

Spread 2 tbsp approx. of pizza sauce on each flatbread, leaving some of the outer edge exposed.

Grate about 15 grams of cheddar on each one and crack a fresh organic egg in the middle of each flatbread.

Place on a baking tray, lined with parchment paper and bake in the oven for 12 minutes.

Remove from the oven and place on a serving plate, drizzle with olive oil, season well with salt and pepper, finally sprinkle with freshly washed rocket.

Enjoy!

Rocket is a peppery bitter detoxifying salad leaf which supports healthy liver function.

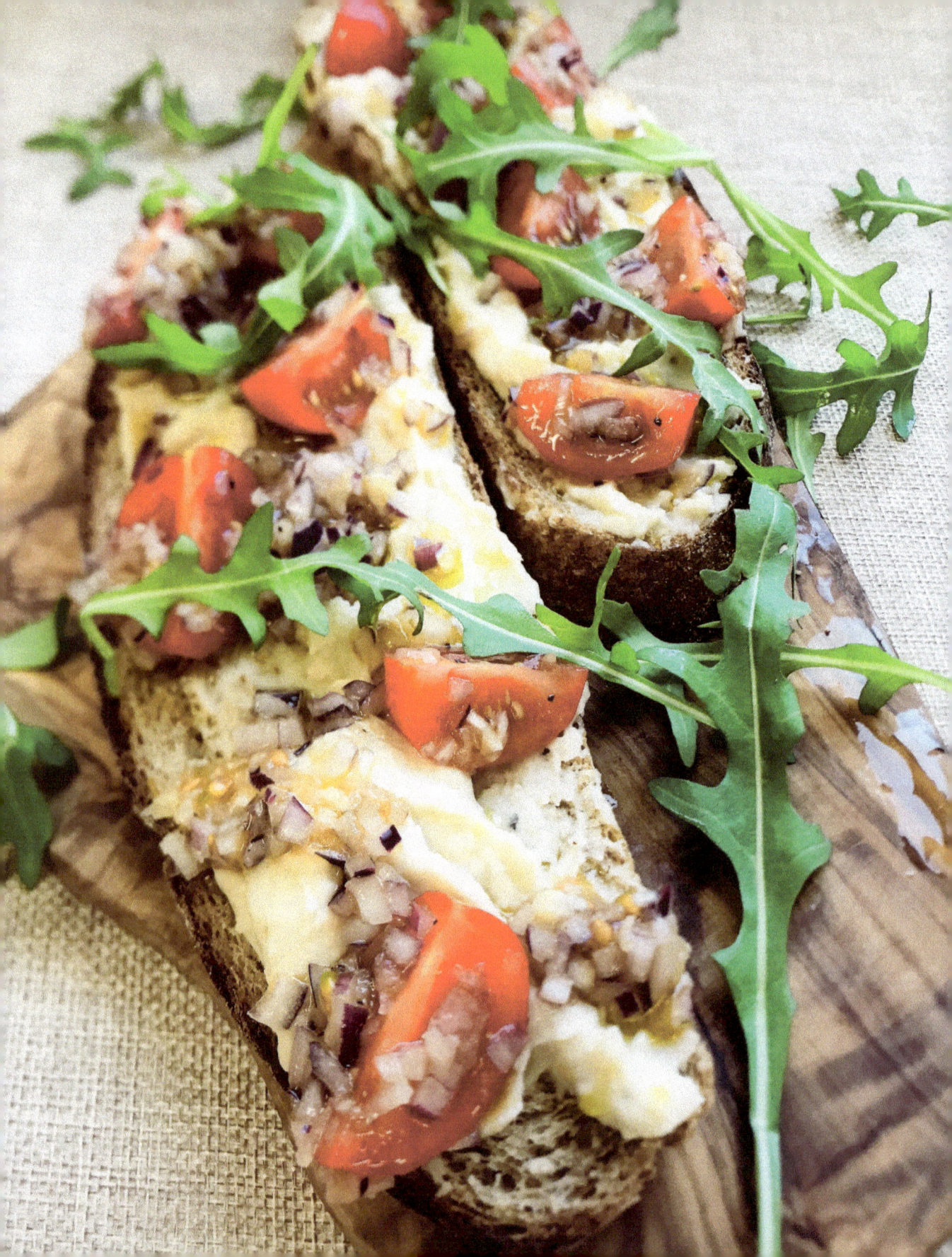

BRUSCHETTA GIGANTI WITH ROASTED GARLIC AND CANNELLINI BUTTER

SERVES 1–2

FOR THE CANNELLINI BUTTER

1 bulb of garlic

240 grams of drained and rinsed cannellini beans (from can)

4 tbsp organic extra virgin olive oil + extra for cooking

Ground Himalayan pink salt

Freshly ground black pepper

FOR THE SALSA

6 cherry tomatoes

1 small red onion

4 tbsp organic extra virgin olive oil

1 clove of garlic

Ground Himalayan pink salt

Freshly ground black pepper

Handful of rocket

Preheat the oven to 200 °C. Cut the bulb of garlic in half, brush with a little olive oil, place in an ovenproof dish, season with salt and pepper and add a splash of water to prevent burning. Roast the garlic for 30 minutes or until soft to touch.

Put the beans, roasted garlic, olive oil and seasoning into a pestle & mortar, bash and mix to a smooth buttery texture.

Finely dice the red onion, chop the garlic with a pinch of salt to form a paste, cut the cherry tomatoes in quarters. Mix together in a bowl with the olive oil and season to taste.

Take 2 large diagonal slices of spelt loaf (SEE PAGE 119) and toast them under the grill, spread with the cannellini butter and top with the salsa and rocket.

Enjoy!

Cannellini beans help you lose weight, regulate blood sugar levels and contribute to a healthy heart.

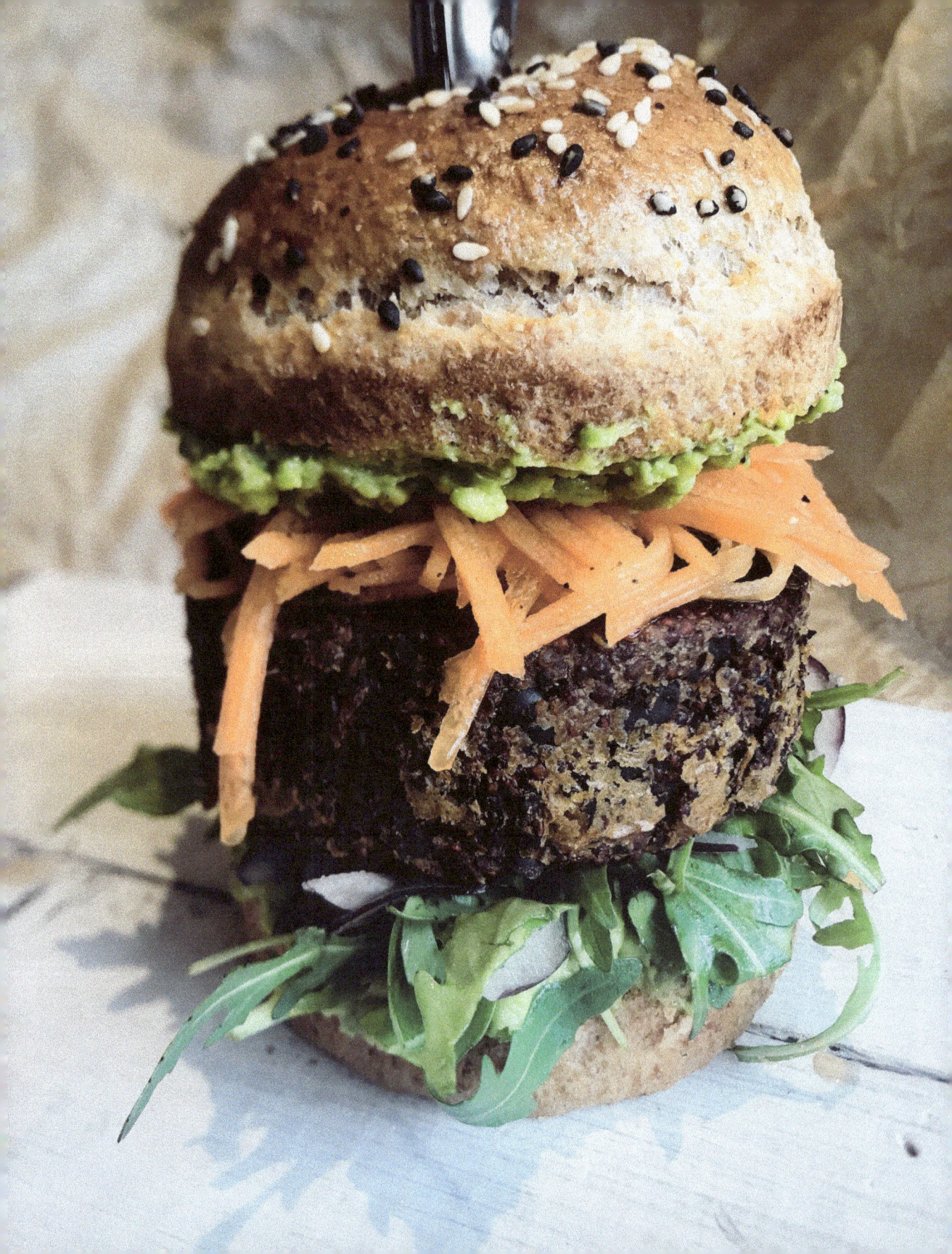

RED QUINOA & BLACKBEAN BURGER

MAKES 3 BURGERS

½ cup red quinoa (soaked in water overnight)

1 ½ cups boiling water

1 tsp organic vegetable bouillon powder

1 can of blackbeans drained and rinsed (235 grams drained weight)

2 tsp harissa paste

1 large egg beaten

2 tbsp wholemeal spelt flour

Ground Himalayan pink salt

Freshly ground black pepper

Organic extra virgin olive oil for cooking

Spelt burger buns (SEE PAGE 113)

1 carrot grated

Juice from ½ orange

1 tbsp pumpkin seeds

Handful of rocket

1 small red onion sliced

1 avocado

Drain the soaked quinoa and place in a medium saucepan with the boiling water and the bouillon. Cook on a high heat, stirring regularly for approx. 14 minutes, or until all the liquid has been absorbed, remove from the heat and cover with a lid and rest for 15 minutes. Meanwhile place the beans in a large mixing bowl and crush with clean hands, until mushy with some texture remaining, add the cooked quinoa to the beans along with the harissa paste, beaten egg and flour, and season well with salt and pepper. Mix thoroughly and place in the fridge for at least 1 hour.

Mix the grated carrot with the orange juice and pumpkin seeds and season well with salt and pepper, set to one side. Mash the avocado with a fork and season well with salt and pepper.

Preheat your oven to 200 °C and put a non-stick frying pan on a high heat. Lightly grease with olive oil, 3, 9 cm diameter, stainless steel cooking rings and place in the pan. Divide your burger mix into 3 equal portions. Put a tsp of olive oil into each ring and spoon in your burger mix, fry for 3 minutes each side and finish in the oven for 15 minutes.

Assemble your burger, cut the burger bun in half and toast under the grill, spread each half with mashed avocado, layer up with rocket & red onion on the bottom followed by the burger, and carrot salad on top, spear with a steak knife and enjoy!

Black beans are a good source of fibre which helps cleanse and protect the colon.

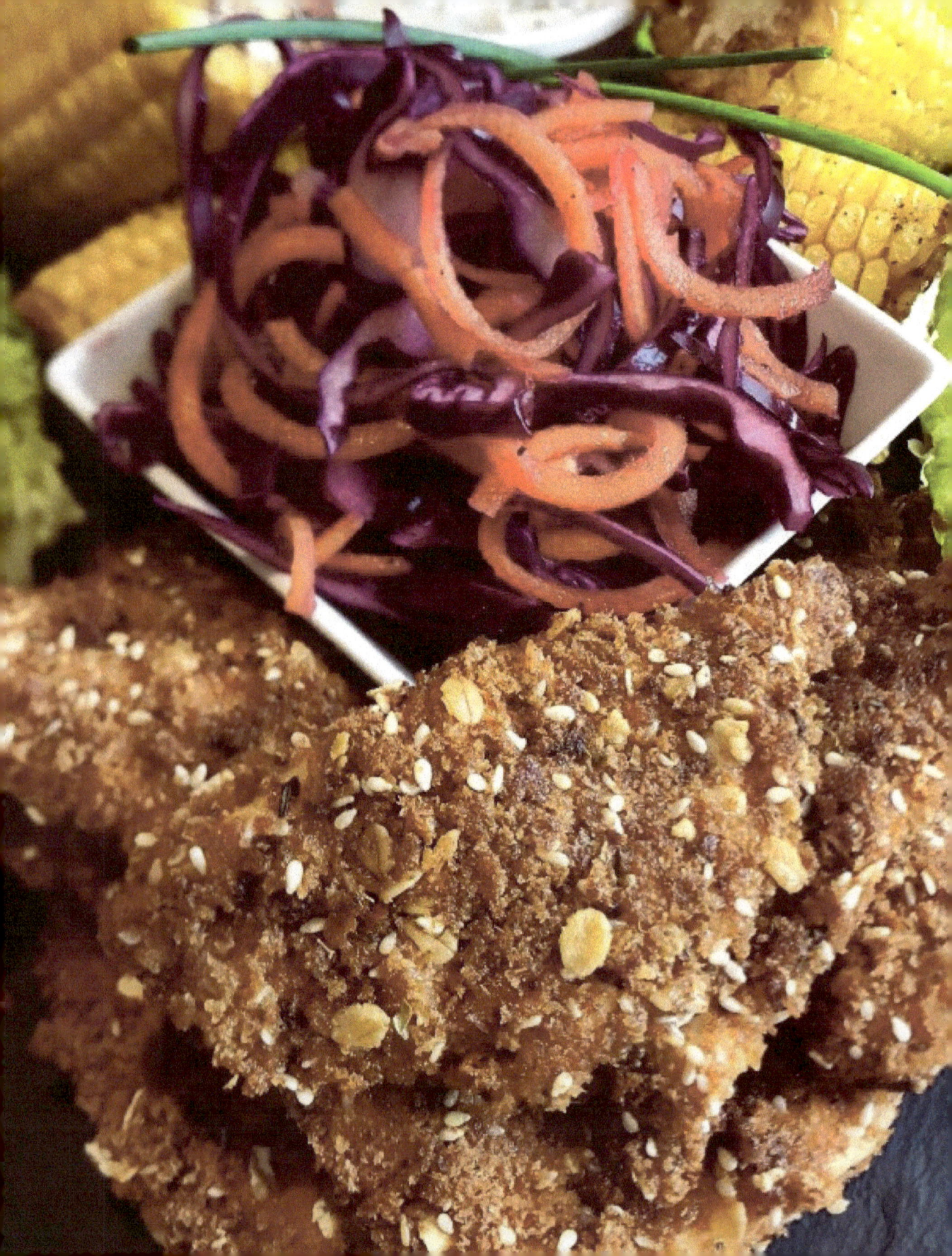

SOUTHERN FRIED CHICKEN

SERVES 2

SECRET SPICE MIX

2 tbsp blackened Cajun spice, 2 tbsp smoked paprika, 2 tbsp garlic granules, 2 tbsp dried oregano & 1 tbsp ground Himalayan pink salt.

SLAW

125 grams shredded carrot, 125 grams shredded red cabbage, 2 tbsp ACV with the mother, ground Himalayan pink salt and freshly ground black pepper.

Mix together the carrot, cabbage, ACV and season well with salt and pepper, cover and place in the fridge.

CHIVE CRÈME FRAICHE

100 mls oat crème fraiche, 10 grams of finely chopped chives, mix and season well with salt and pepper.

ROAST 4 ORGANIC MINI CORN COBS

in a preheated oven 200 °C for 20 minutes, with a drizzle of olive oil and salt and pepper.

GARNISH

baby gem leaves and vine tomato wedges.

FOR THE CHICKEN

300 grams organic chicken breast
250 grams of spelt loaf
(SEE PAGE 119)
½ cup wholemeal spelt flour
2 organic eggs
2 tbsp sesame seeds
2 tbsp of jumbo organic oats

Cut the loaf into chunks and put in the food processor, along with 1 tbsp of the spice mix and blitz into fine breadcrumbs, transfer to a large mixing bowl and add the sesame seeds and oats, thoroughly mix until seeds and oats are well distributed, place half of this into a food bag and freeze for another time. Put the spelt flour in another bowl and thoroughly mix 1 tbsp of spice mix into it. Crack the 2 eggs into a third bowl and add 1 tbsp of the spice mix and a splash of water, whisk thoroughly until smooth. Trim and cut the chicken into large goujons, place in the spiced flour and coat well, shake off access and place in the egg mixture, mix and ensure chicken in completely coated in the egg. Leave the chicken in the egg mixture for 10 minutes to allow the flavour to develop, now take each goujon and place in the breadcrumbs. Make sure the chicken has an even coat of breadcrumbs before transferring to a plate and chill in the fridge for 10 minutes.

Meanwhile get your large non-stick frying pan on a high heat, and your oven to 200 °C. Pour in a drizzle of olive oil, and carefully place your goujons in the pan. Fry for 1–2 minutes each side and transfer to a baking tray and place in the oven for 10–12 minutes.

Assemble and enjoy!

Sweetcorn promotes a healthy digestive tract.

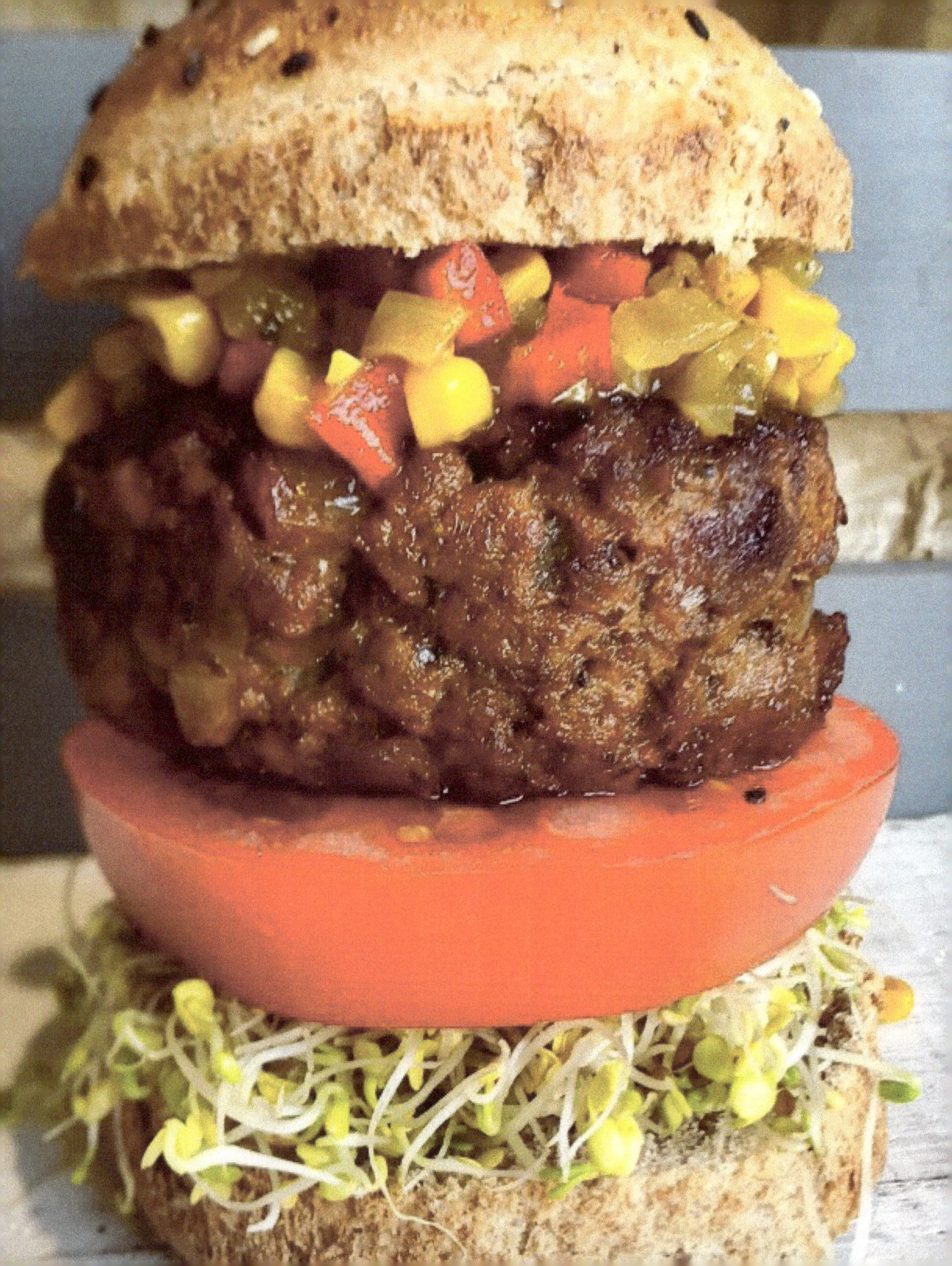

PROPER BEEF BURGER

MAKES 4 BURGERS

500 grams organic grass fed minced beef (from chuck) with 15% fat

1 medium sized onion

2 cloves garlic

1 organic beef stock cube

1 tbsp dried oregano

70 grams tomato puree

1 litre boiling water

1 tbsp organic extra virgin olive oil

Peel and finely chop the onion and mince the garlic, heat a large non-stick frying pan and sauté the onions & garlic for a few minutes, pour in the boiling water, add stock cube, add oregano and tomato puree, this needs to boil and reduce until almost all the liquid has evaporated, it takes 30-45 minutes, keep an eye on it and stir regularly. (Ideally make this the day before and refrigerate.) With clean hands thoroughly mix the cold flavouring paste with the burger mince, divide into 4 balls, compact with your hands and place in a 9 cm stainless steel cooking ring to achieve a nice round shaped burger.

SWEETCORN RELISH

2 cans organic sweetcorn (320 grams)

1 tbsp organic extra virgin olive oil

2 cloves garlic

1 medium sized onion

1 red pepper

1 tsp curry powder

4 tbsp raw organic honey

1 cup hot water

Ground Himalayan pink salt

Freshly ground black pepper

Peel and finely chop the onion, dice the red pepper, mince the garlic. Place a large non-stick frying pan on a high heat, sauté the onions, garlic and pepper in the olive oil for 5 minutes, stirring regularly, add the corn, the water, curry powder and honey, season well with salt and pepper. Reduce until most of the liquid has evaporated and becomes syrupy. Place in a sterilised jar with a clasped lid & seal, leave open until completely cool, close and place in the fridge. (Make this well in advance, it keeps very well in the fridge for 5+ days.)

OTHER INGREDIENTS, SUPER SPROUTED SEEDS, BEEF TOMATO, SPELT BURGER BUNS (SEE PAGE 113)

Preheat your oven to 200 °C. Pan fry the burgers (in their cooking rings) in a large non-stick frying pan for 2 minutes each side, with a little olive oil, on a high heat, and season with a little salt & pepper. Transfer to a baking tray and cook in the oven for 20–25 minutes until fully cooked all the way through.

Build your burger – toast your spelt bun and layer up with sprouted seeds, sliced beef tomato, the juicy burger, topped with some sweetcorn relish...

Enjoy!

Organic grass-fed beef is an excellent source of high quality protein, iron and omega-3 fatty acids

"SPAG BOL"

Puy Lentil and Butternut Squash Bolognese with Blackbean Spaghetti

MAKES 5–6 PORTIONS

1 cup of dried puy (green) lentils soaked in plenty of cold water overnight

1 red onion finely diced

1 green pepper finely diced

5 chestnut mushrooms chopped finely

3 ribs celery finely diced

1 carrot peeled and finely diced

2 cloves garlic minced with a little Himalayan salt

600 grams peeled and diced butternut squash

140 grams tomato puree

2 tbsp organic veg bouillon powder

1 litre boiling water

1 tbsp extra virgin organic olive oil

1 tbsp dried oregano

2 large sprig of fresh rosemary

Ground Himalayan pink salt

Freshly ground black pepper

200 grams organic dried blackbean spaghetti (there are plenty of other alternatives pastas on the market)

Sundried focaccia bread (SEE PAGE 111)

Organic grass-fed garlic butter (optional)

Place a large stainless steel saucepan on a high heat, add the olive oil followed by the onions, garlic, celery, carrot, green pepper, mushrooms, oregano and rosemary, cook for a few minutes then add the hot water along with the veg bouillon. Bring to the boil and simmer for 10 minutes, now add the lentils and squash and simmer for a further 10 minutes or until the lentils and squash are tender, add the tomato puree and season with the salt and pepper, mix thoroughly and simmer for 5 more minutes.

Meanwhile cook the spaghetti (according to pack instructions) in plenty of boiling salted water for 46 minutes and refresh in cold water to halt the cooking process.

Cut the focaccia bread into triangles and spread with garlic butter (optional) and toast under a hot grill.

Keep your Bolognese and spaghetti separate until you wish to eat it, reheat the required amount in a pan with a splash of water to prevent drying out, serve with toasted garlic focaccia.

Enjoy!

Butternut Squash has a wide range of nutrients including beta carotene and magnesium which support cardiovascular health.

CITRUS SALMON PATE WITH PICKLED FENNEL SALAD AND FOCACCIA TOASTS

FOR THE PATE

350 grams salmon (preferably the belly meat)

200 mls oat crème fraiche

Juice from ½ lemon

Juice from ½ lime

Juice from ½ orange

2 heaped tbsp. of chopped dill

Ground Himalayan pink salt

Freshly ground black pepper

Poach the salmon in seasoned water and drain, allow to cool and place in the food processor with the crème fraiche & dill, season very well, turn on the machine and pour in the citrus juice whilst on, blitz until very smooth, taste and adjust the seasoning as required.

FOR THE PICKLED FENNEL

1 fennel bulb

500 mls boiling water

2 tbsp apple cider vinegar (with the mother culture)

1 tbsp raw organic honey

1 tbsp ground Himalayan pink salt

1 cinnamon stick

1 segmented orange

Organic extra virgin olive oil

Add the vinegar, honey, salt and cinnamon stick to the boiling water and stir well. Finely slice the fennel bulb and place in a large jar, pour over the hot pickle solution and leave to cool. Once cool, cover and place in the fridge overnight. Drain the fennel and drizzle with olive oil and mix in the orange segments.

For the focaccia toast, take out a chunk of sundried tomato focaccia bread (SEE PAGE 111) from the freezer, slice thinly and toast in a hot non-stick frying pan with a little olive oil.

Serve up and enjoy!

Essential omega-3 fats are concentrated in the belly of the salmon

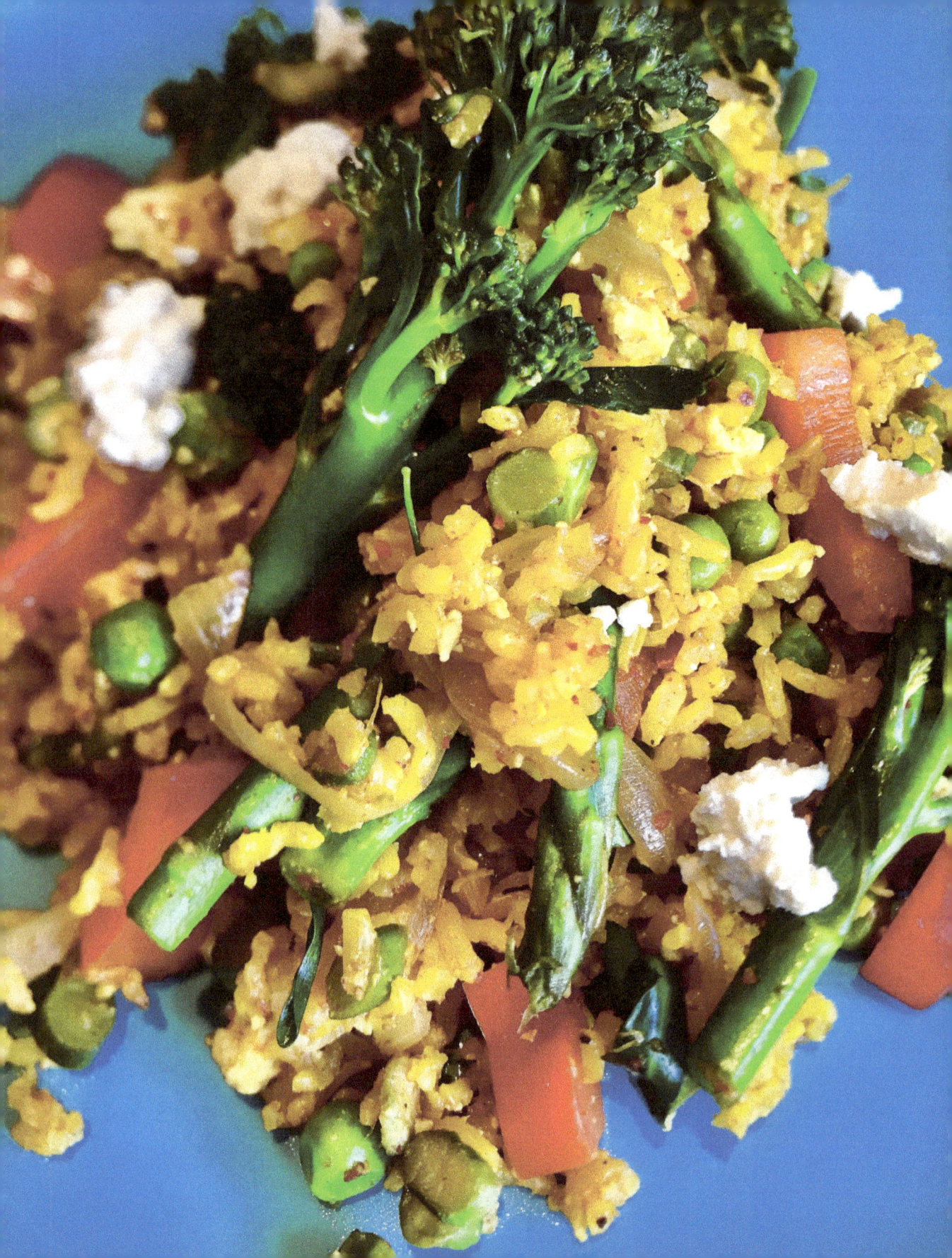

SINGAPORE FRIED RICE WITH SCRAMBLED TOFU

SERVES 2–3

1 cup of brown basmati rice (soaked in water overnight)

1 tsp organic vegetable bouillon powder

1 tsp turmeric powder

150 grams organic tofu

2 tsp madras curry paste (store bought)

1 medium onion

1 red pepper

100 grams asparagus

100 grams tender stem broccoli

50 grams frozen peas

1 tsp Korean red pepper flakes

Ground Himalayan pink salt

Freshly ground black pepper

1 tbsp organic extra virgin olive oil

Rinse off the rice and place in a large saucepan, add the vegetable bouillon and turmeric and pour in 1 litre of boiling water, boil for 20–22 minutes, adding a little extra boiling water if required. Drain the rice and leave to steam off.

Meanwhile, peel and slice the onion, wash and slice the pepper, finely chop the stems of the asparagus and broccoli, leaving the tips intact.

Place a non-stick wok on a high heat and fry the onion with the olive oil for a good 10 minutes, stirring continuously to prevent burning, add the pepper, asparagus, broccoli, peas, curry paste and pepper flakes. Add a splash of hot water and steam fry for 5 minutes. When all liquid has evaporated add the warm rice, and season well with your salt and pepper, toss and stir until everything is evenly distributed, taste and adjust seasoning as required.

Finally break the tofu with your fingertips and crumble into the rice mixture, stir well and serve up.

Enjoy!

Turmeric contains potent anti-inflammatory, anti-oxidant compounds, which protect against free radical damage.

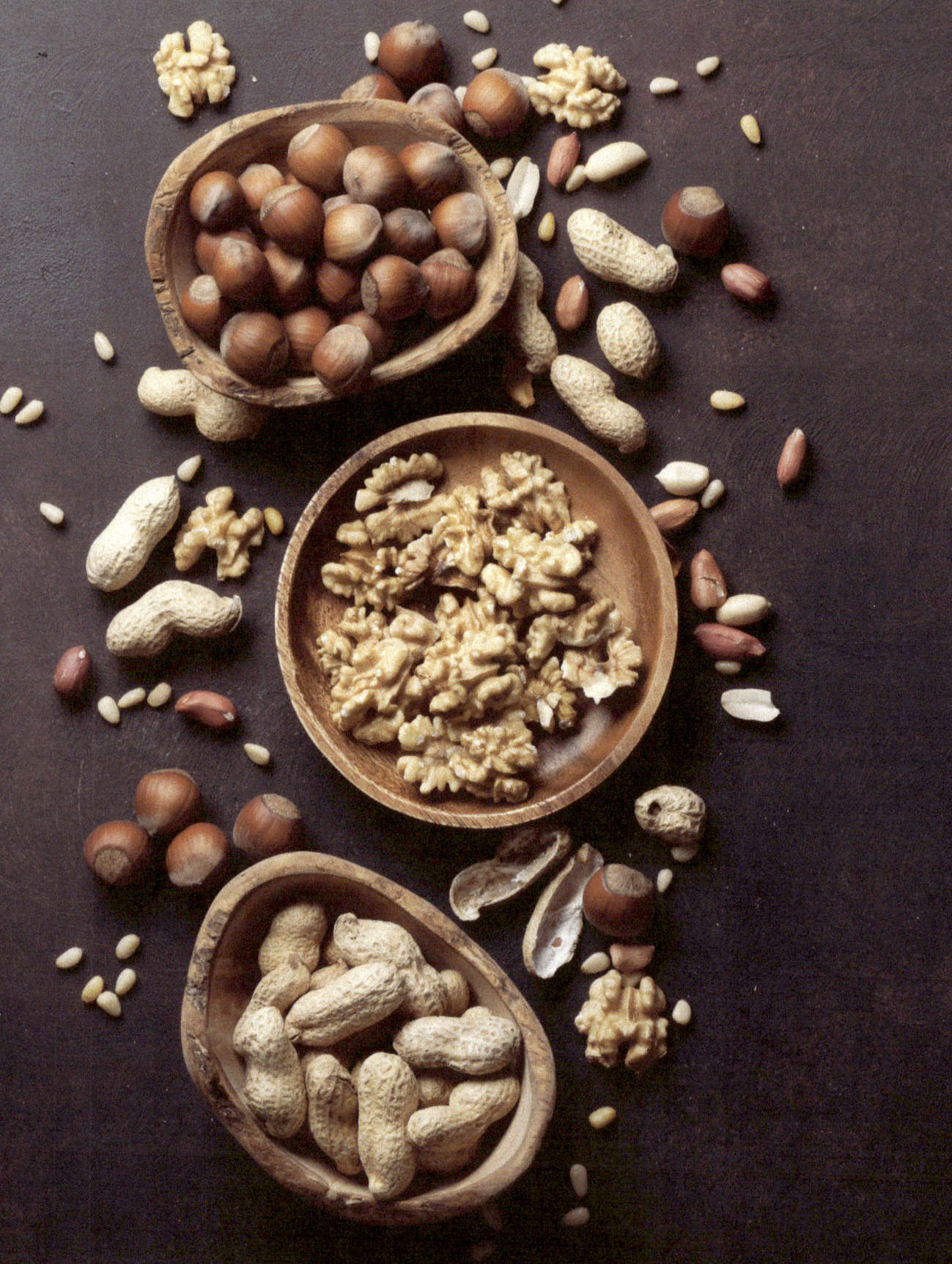

HEALTHY SNACKS

Simple snack ideas can be ; a piece of fruit, handful of mixed nuts, oatcakes with nutbutter, half a smoothie, etc., etc... However, you can really make it a lot more interesting by preparing some of the following, nutritious recipes in advance.

The sweet ones can be used as a dessert too!

FIRE ROASTED RED PEPPER AND MINT HUMMUS WITH CRUDITES

SERVES 2

240 grams of rinsed canned chickpeas

2 fire roasted red peppers (store bought jar)

handful of mint leaves

1 tbsp tahini

The juice of 1 lemon

3 tbsp olive oil

1 small carrot (peeled)

1 rib of celery (washed)

½ green pepper

½ yellow pepper

½ cucumber

For the Hummus, I use a nutribullet, however any blender will do the job.

Place chickpeas, roast peppers, mint, tahini, lemon juice and olive oil in the large nutribullet cup and blend until smooth.

Cut the carrot, celery, green pepper, yellow pepper and cucumber into small sticks.

Serve hummus in a small dish with crudités on the side.

Tahini is made from sesame seeds, a great source of vitamin E which supports heart health, skin condition and the nervous system.

RICE CRISPY BARS

MAKES 22 BARS APPROX.

300 grams of jumbo raw peanuts (soaked overnight in water)

Pinch of Himalayan salt

450 grams pitted Medjool dates

100 grams organic sugar free puffed wholegrain rice

2 tbsp chia seeds

2 tbsp Maca powder

¾ cup date syrup

½ cup coconut oil

Put peanuts in the food processor with the pinch of salt and blitz until you achieve a peanut butter texture (takes about 5 minutes, you'll need to stop it a few times to scrape down the sides). Gently melt the coconut oil and carefully add it to the peanut butter along with the date syrup & Maca powder, blitz again until well incorporated. Transfer this mixture to a very large mixing bowl.

Now put the dates into the food processor and blitz until they become a sticky ball.

Add the dates to the peanut butter along with the puffed rice & chia seeds.

Using clean hands, mix everything together thoroughly, and press into a greaseproof paper lined traybake tin (320 mm × 220 mm). Chill for at least 1 hour in the fridge.

Turn out onto a large chopping board and cut into snack size bars.

Coconut oil can boost your immune system, it has antibacterial, antifungal and antiviral properties.

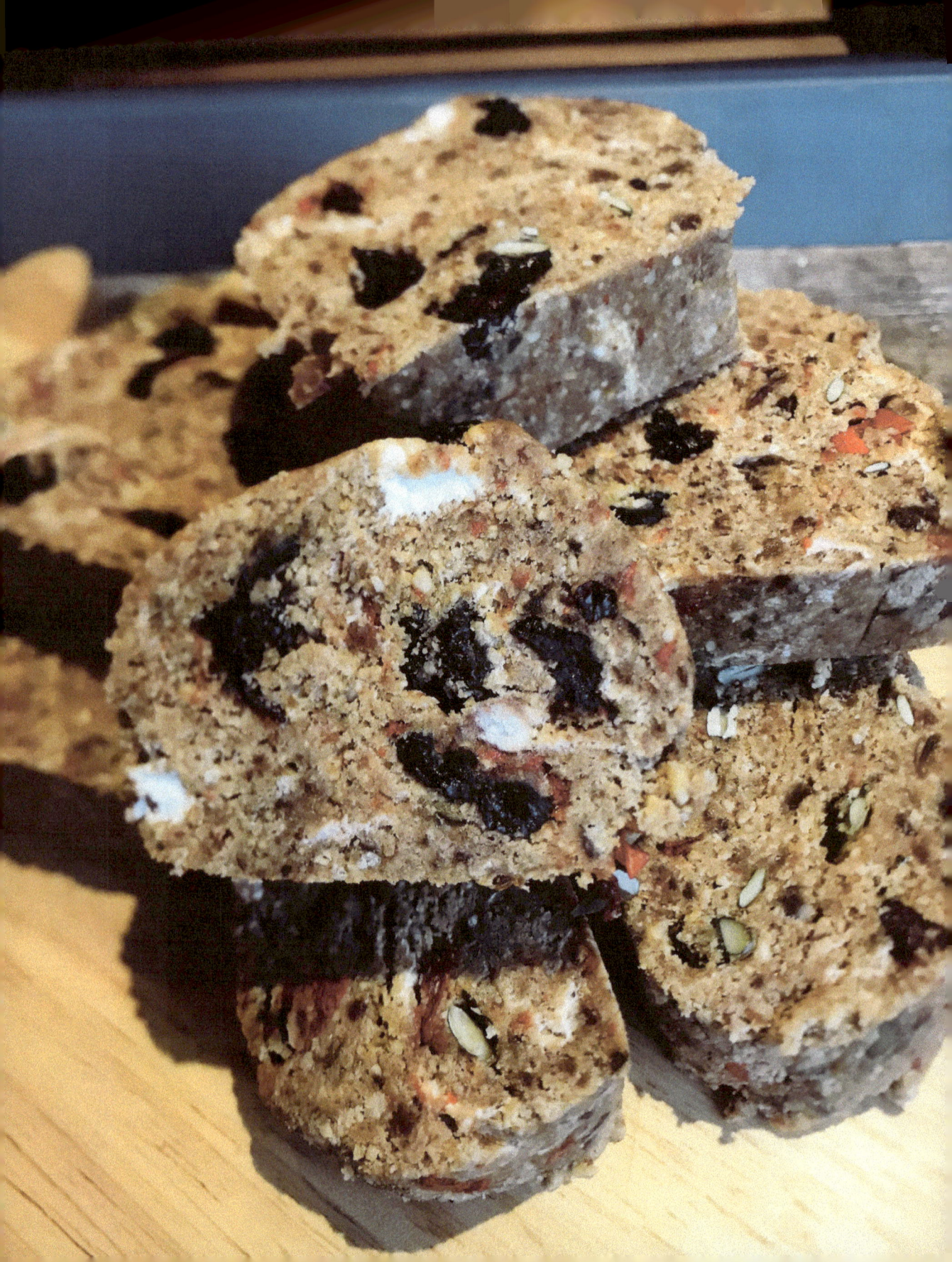

MAKES ABOUT 18 CAKES

Whilst this recipe is based on the classic flavours of the famous "fifteens" traybake, the numbers are amped up significantly.

28 organic oatcakes

450 grams pitted Medjool dates

90 grams dried cherries

50 grams goji berries

¼ cup coconut oil

¼ cup date syrup

50 grams pumpkin seeds (soaked in water for 2 hours)

2 tbsp Maca powder

75 grams of sugar free marshmallows (made with beef gelatin) (optional)

Soak the dried cherries and goji berries in hot water for 10 mins, then drain and leave to one side.

Put oatcakes in a food processor and blitz to a crumb, gently melt the coconut oil in a small saucepan and add to the biscuit crumb along with the date syrup and blitz again until well mixed, then transfer this mixture into a very large mixing bowl.

Now put the dates in the food processor (no need to wash it) and blitz until they form a sticky ball, add them to the biscuit crumb along with the drained cherries & goji berries, pumpkin seeds, Maca powder and marshmallows (if you choose to use them).

Using clean hands, mix everything together until you achieve a pliable cookie dough texture.

Roll the mixture into a log in a large sheet of grease proof paper. Remove from paper and slice into 15 mm slices (½ inch).

Pumpkin seeds are high in zinc, they are useful for promoting men's fertility and prostate health. They are also a good source of B vitamins and magnesium to support energy levels and stress management.

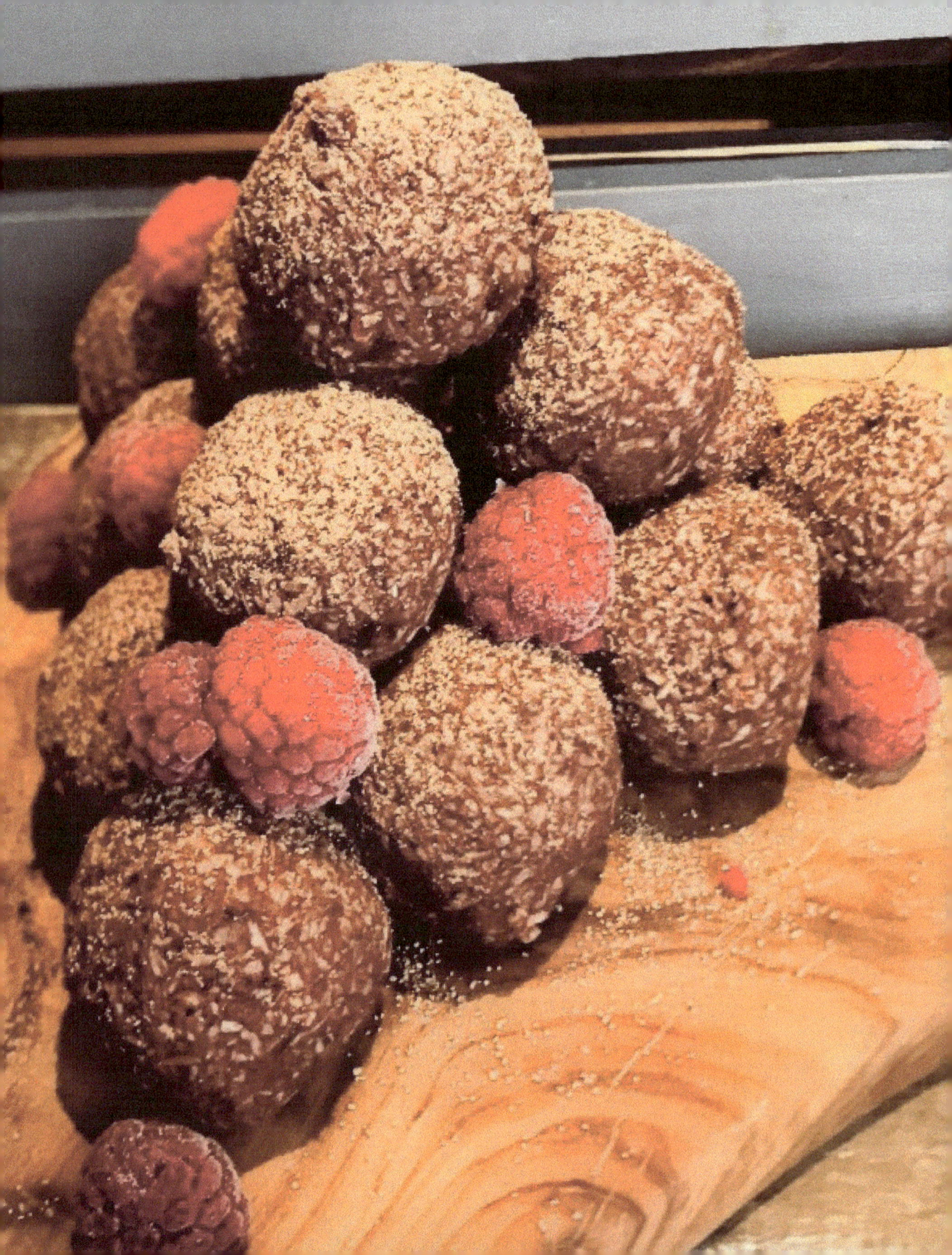

DECADENT RASPBERRY RUFFLES

MAKES 35 RUFFLES

350 grams desiccated coconut

350 grams pitted Medjool dates

200 grams frozen raspberries

3 tbsp organic local raw honey

2 tsp vanilla bean paste

2 tbsp chia seeds

4 tbsp cacao powder

Put dates into a food processor, followed by half of the coconut, the raspberries, cacao powder, vanilla bean paste, chia seeds & honey. Blitz to a paste.

You will notice at this stage the paste is a little wet. Transfer the paste to a large mixing bowl and add the other half of the coconut.

Using clean hands mix thoroughly, this will achieve the correct consistency to roll the mix into ruffles.

Use the palms of your hands in a circular motion to shape the ruffles.

Dates are high in potassium, an essential mineral that maintains proper muscle contractions, including those of the heart.

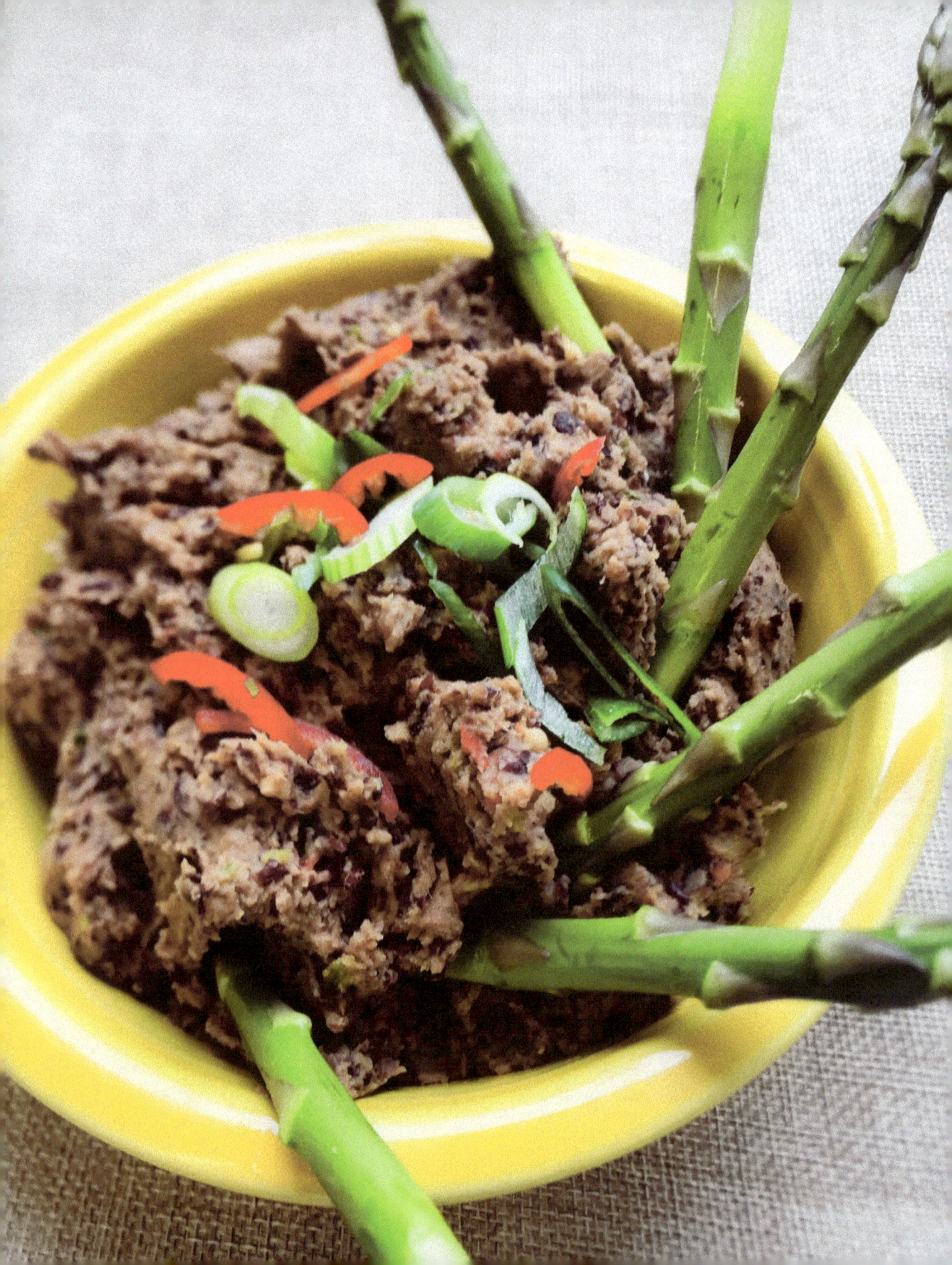

ASIAN KIDNEY BEAN DIP WITH CRUNCHY ASPARAGUS SOLDIERS

480 grams from can, drained & rinsed kidney beans

1 red chilli

2 cloves garlic

3 spring onions

1 thumb size piece of ginger

1 tbsp red Thai curry paste (shop bought) (contains shrimp paste)

Ground Himalayan pink salt

Freshly ground black pepper

125 grams asparagus spears

Prepare the asparagus, removing woody end if necessary (however most vegetable retailers will have this already done) and peel of a little of the outer edge at the bottom of the spear, place in cold water until ready for use.

Deseed and finely chop red chilli, crush the garlic, peel and finely chop the ginger, wash and finely chop spring onions.

Put the kidney beans into a food processor, add the chilli , garlic, ginger, spring onion & curry paste. Season well with your salt and pepper. Pulse the mixture until a semi smooth consistency is achieved, to retain a little texture (you may need to stop and scrape down the sides a few times).

Serve with your crunchy asparagus soldiers.

Recipe keeps well in the fridge for at least 3 days.

Garlic supports heart health, immunity and good circulation.

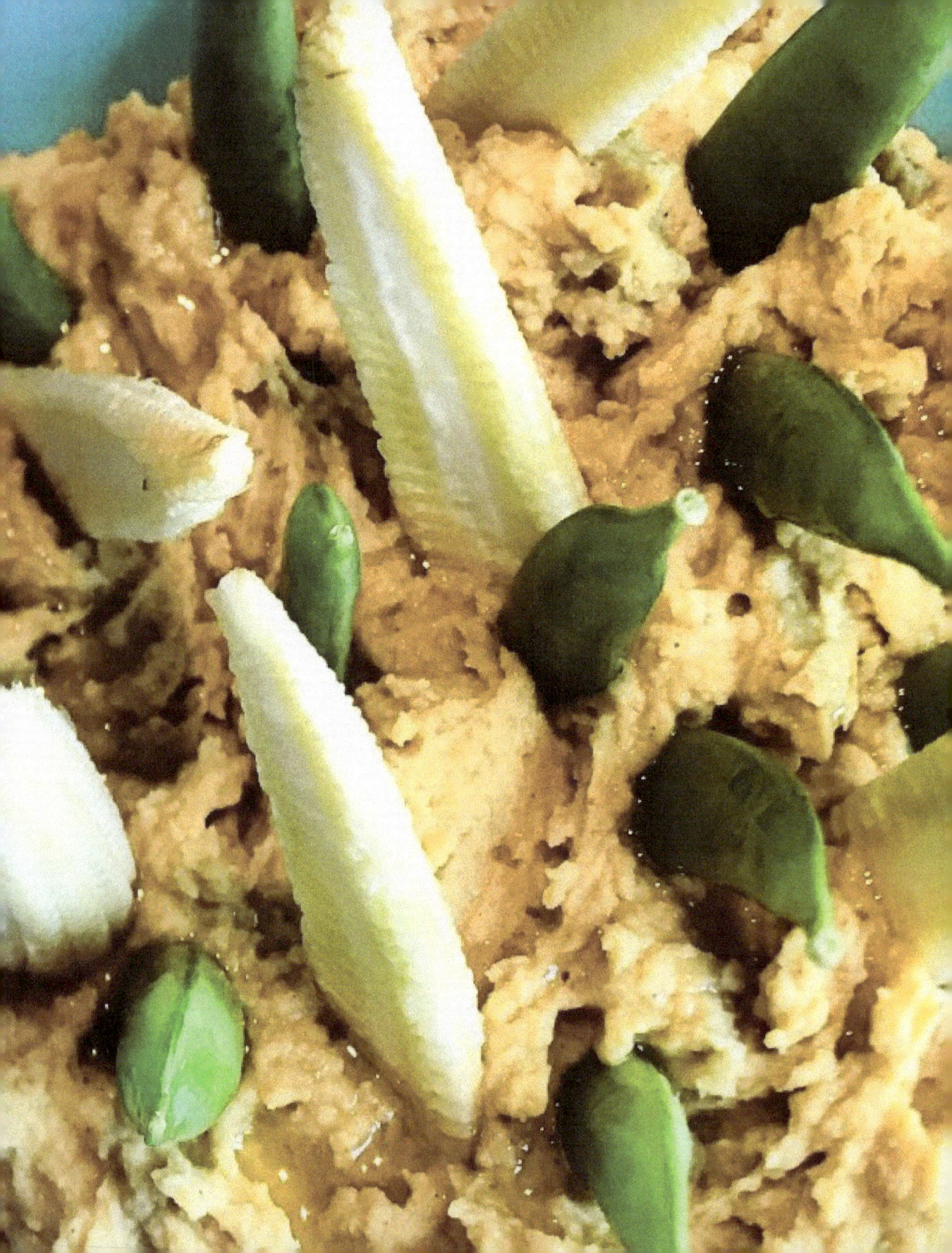

CURRIED BUTTER BEAN DIP WITH CRUNCHY SUGAR SNAPS AND BABY CORN

470 grams (from can) organic butter beans, drained and rinsed

2 tsp good quality madras curry paste (shop bought)

Ground Himalayan pink salt

2 tbsp extra virgin olive oil

100 mls water

Fresh sugar snap peas

Fresh baby corn

Put the butter beans in the food processor, add the curry paste, water & only 1 tbsp of olive oil, season with Himalayan salt (remember you can always add but you can't take away with seasoning, start with a little and taste, repeat until your happy with the balance).

Wash the sugar snaps and baby corn in cold water and serve with the dip, drizzle with the remaining olive oil.

Sugar snap peas are high in fibre and vitamin C which supports a healthy digestive and immune systems.

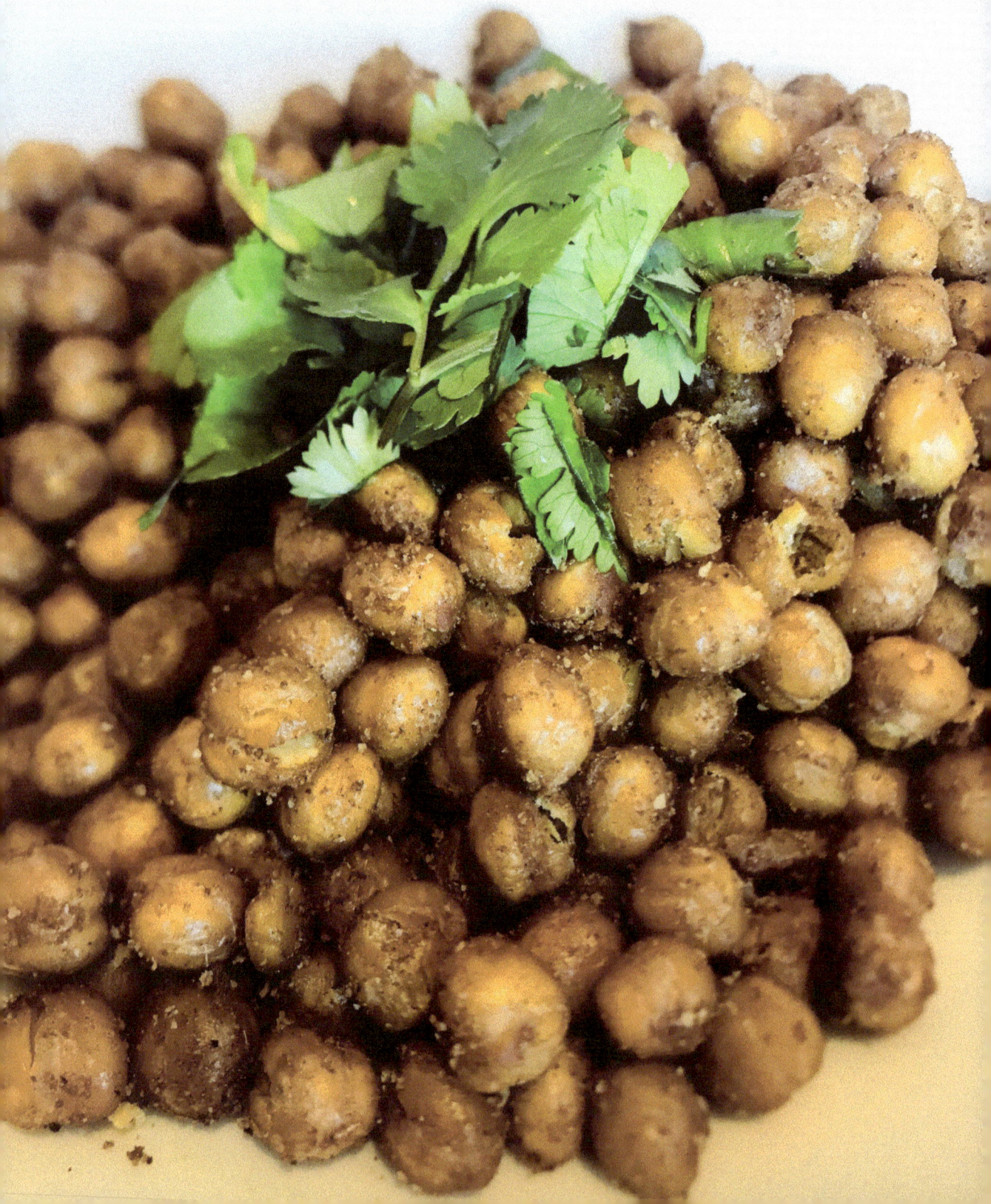

CUMIN ROASTED CHICKPEAS

460 grams (drained weight) organic chickpeas rinsed

2 tsp ground cumin

2 tbsp extra virgin olive oil

Ground Himalayan pink salt

Preheat your oven to 200 °C.

Dry the chickpeas on a clean tea towel and transfer to a mixing bowl.

Add the cumin & olive oil and lightly season with salt. Give the chickpeas a good stir to ensure the oil and seasonings have evenly coated them.

Place on a greaseproof paper lined baking tray and roast in the oven for 22–25 minutes. You will hear them start to pop towards the end of the cooking time, this is an indicator that they are almost ready.

Remove from the oven and allow to cool and enjoy.

Cumin is rich in powerful anti-inflammatory antioxidants

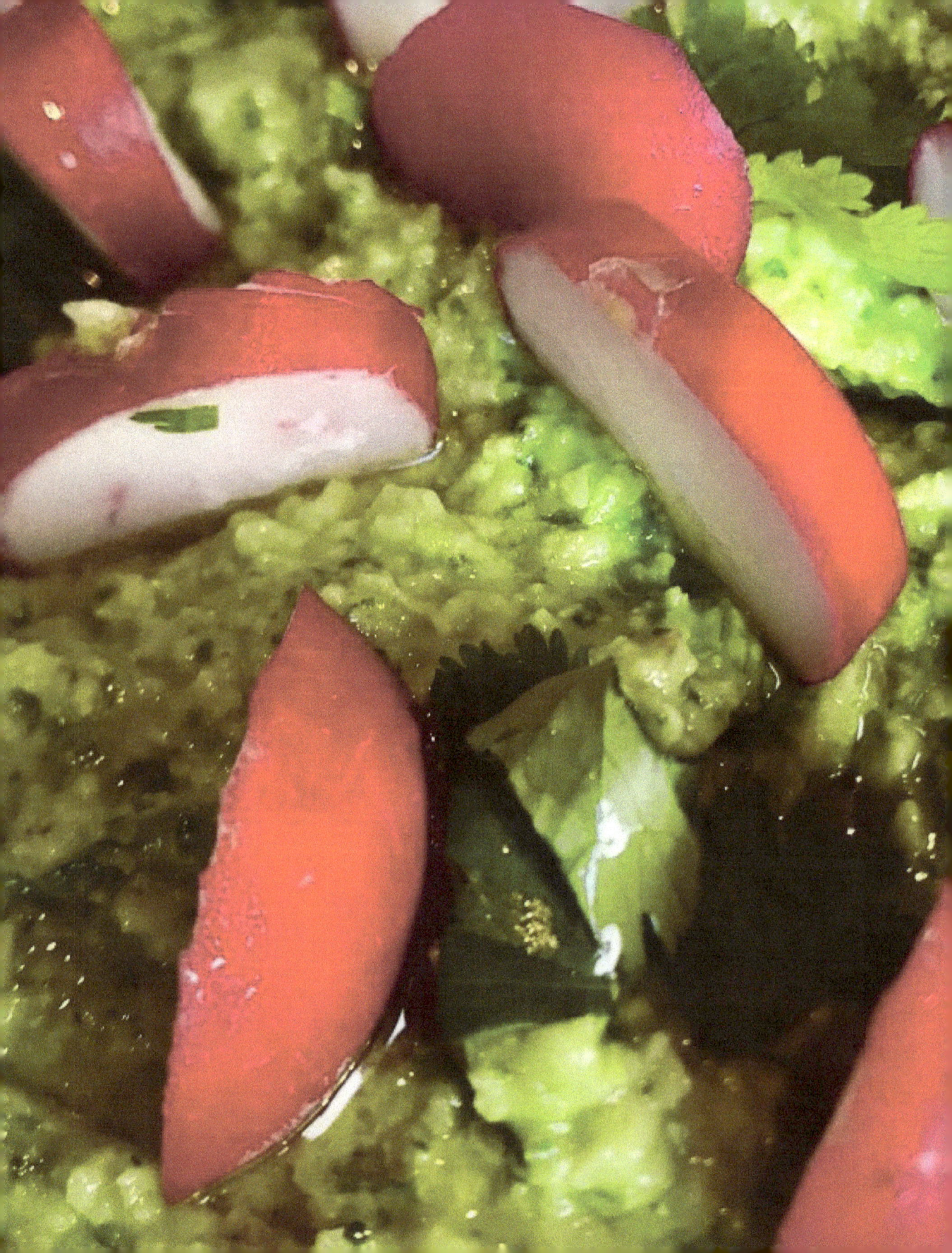

BROAD BEAN GUACAMOLE WITH CRUNCHY RADISHES

380 grams frozen broad beans

1 medium ripe avocado

50 grams coriander

Juice of 1 lime

Ground Himalayan pink salt

100 mls water

2 tbsp organic extra virgin olive oil

Fresh radishes

Defrost the broad beans under cold running water.

Put the broad beans in the food processor, scoop out the flesh of the avocado and finely chop the coriander and add both to the broad beans. Pour in the lime juice and water, lightly season with salt. Blitz the mixture until smooth, however some texture will remain.

Wash and slice the radishes. Serve the guacamole in a dish and drizzle with olive oil.

Broad beans are high in plant protein, they are also nutrient dense, providing an array of vitamins and minerals.

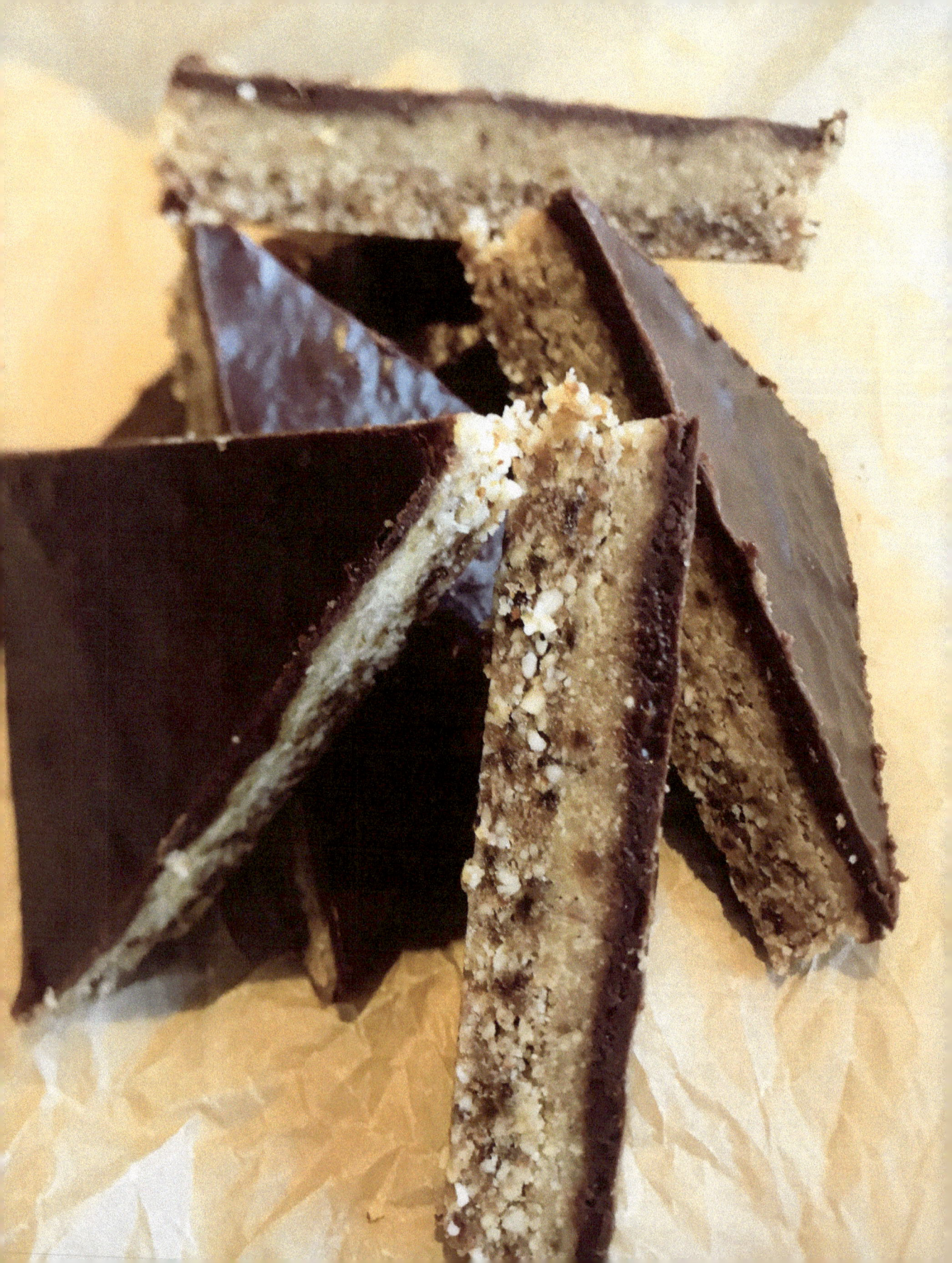

MILLIONAIRES SHORTBREAD

MAKES 12 SQUARES OR 24 TRIANGLES

FOR THE BASE

250 grams raw almonds

250 grams pitted dates

Put the almonds in the food processor and blitz to a breadcrumb texture, add the dates, blitz again until well blended. Grease & line a 320 mm × 220 mm traybake tray with greaseproof paper, ensuring the paper comes up the sides, and press the mixture into the tray, ensuring even distribution into the corners and sides, set to one side.

FOR THE CARAMEL

250 grams cashew nuts

½ cup of melted coconut oil

130 grams pitted dates

2 tsp organic vanilla bean paste

Put the cashew nuts into the food processor and blitz to a fine crumb, add the coconut oil, dates & vanilla bean paste, continue to blitz until a smooth sticky caramel texture is achieved. Spread this mixture on top of the base, once again ensuring evenness , Its best to use your fingertips for this bit. Now place the tray flat in the freezer whilst you make the chocolate layer.

FOR THE CHOCOLATE LAYER

1/3 cup melted coconut oil

2 tbsp cacao powder

¼ cup organic local raw honey

Place the coconut oil, honey & cacao powder into a bowl and whisk together to a smooth consistency. Pour this on top of the caramel layer, tilting in all directions until the chocolate has evenly coated the entire surface. Place in the fridge for at least 2 hours before removing from tray and cutting into your preferred shapes.

Enjoy!

Almonds are a good source of the minerals, zinc, magnesium and potassium and are very rich in vitamin E, which supports the brain, cardiovascular and respiratory systems.

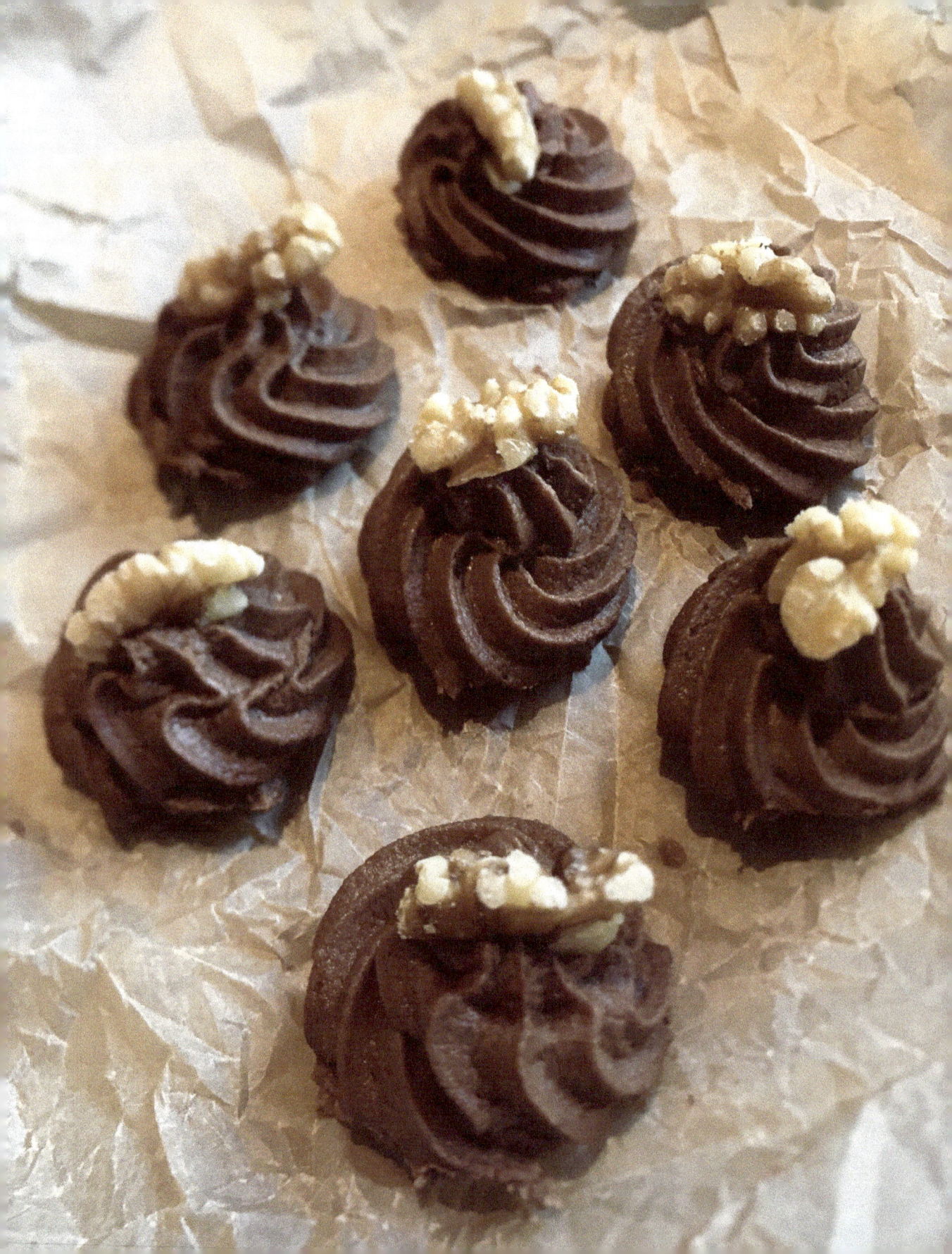

WALNUT WHIP

MAKES 18 APPROX.

1 medium ripe avocado

1 ripe banana

200 grams pitted Medjool dates

200 grams walnuts + more for garnish

2 tbsp cacao powder

80 mls water

Scoop out the flesh of the avocado and put in the food processor along with the banana, dates, walnuts, cacao powder & water.

Blitz for a good 10 minutes, stopping to scrape down the sides as necessary, until you achieve a very thick but smooth texture.

Spoon the mixture into a large piping bag with a wide fluted nozzle.

Line a tray with greaseproof paper and pipe little rosettes until all the mixture is done and garnish with bits of leftover walnuts.

Refrigerate for at least 2 hours to set and then transfer to the freezer. This recipe is best served from the freezer as the avocado and banana will quickly turn.

Enjoy!

Cacao is very high in antioxidants which helps protect against free radical damage.

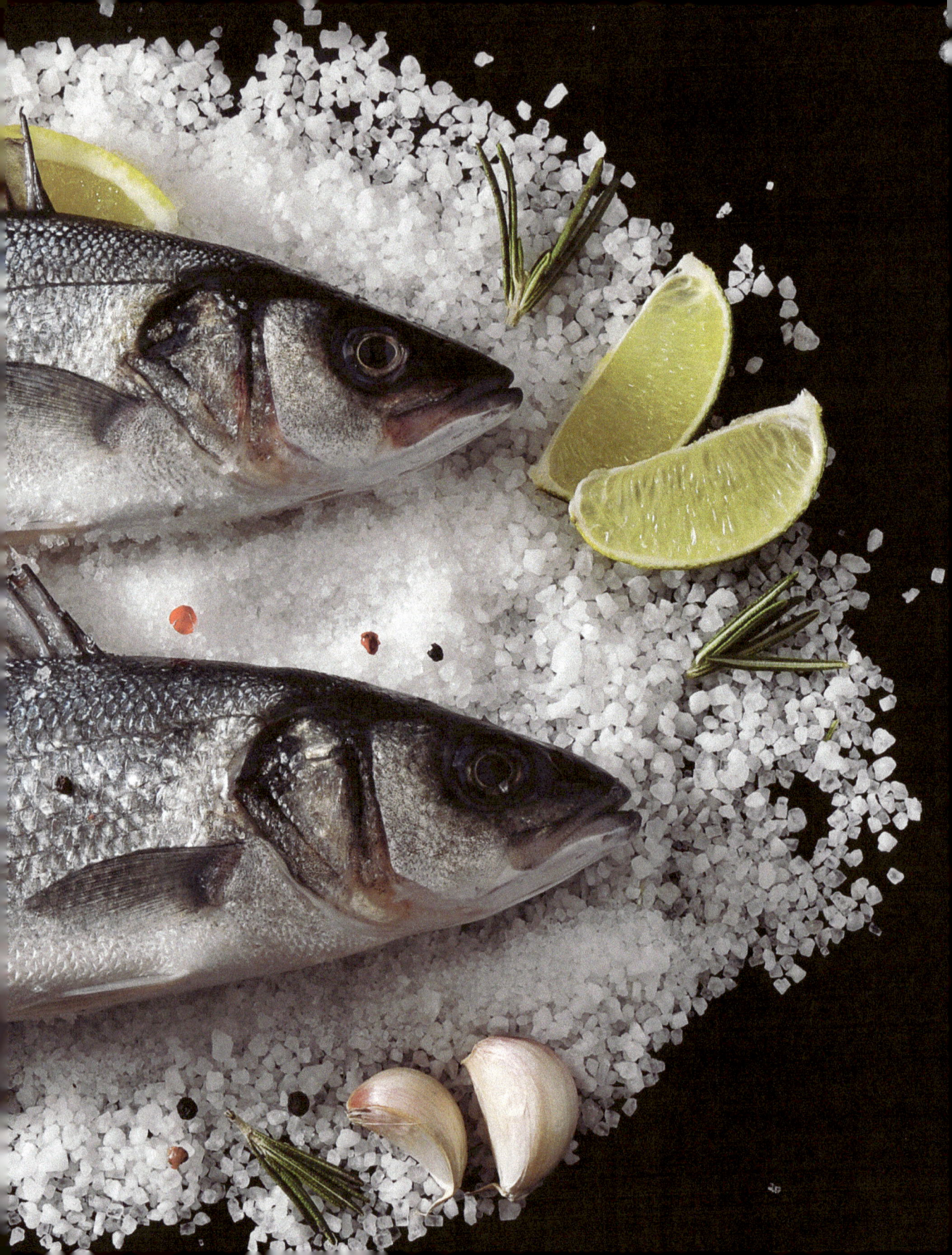

PROPER DINNERS

The main event, the one you look forward to all day, and also the one you don't want to slave over.

Some of the following recipes are a healthy twist on classic dishes we all love as a treat or takeaway. Now you can enjoy your favourites, guilt free. There are also some original vegan meals too, which everyone can enjoy.

I would recommend eating 2 vegan dinners per week, even for non-vegan/vegetarians, to pack in more plant protein.

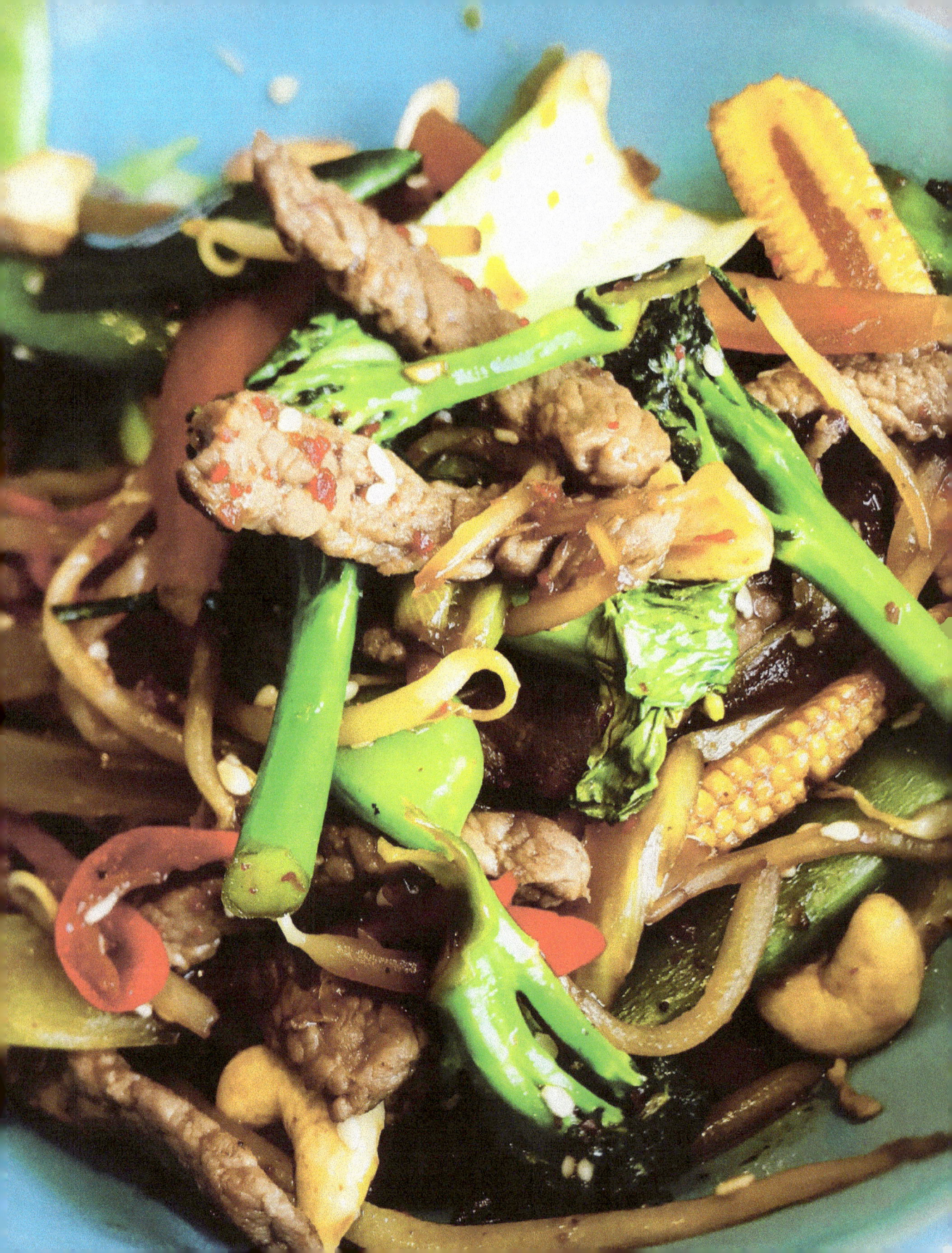

HONEY CHILLI BEEF STIR-FRY

SERVES 1

1 Small organic grass-fed sirloin steak (visible fat removed and finely sliced)

1 tbsp organic extra virgin olive oil

5 mange tout

5 snap peas

2 florets of stem broccoli (split into strands)

1 pak choi (core removed)

½ carrot (thinly sliced)

½ rib of celery (thinly slice)

1 spring onion (finely sliced)

1 red chilli (finely sliced)

2 baby corn (halved long ways)

handful of beansprouts

Small handful of cashew nuts (toasted)

½ tsp sesame seeds

2 tbsp organic raw honey

2 tbsp light soy sauce

½ tsp Korean red pepper flakes

Place a large non-stick frying pan on a high heat. When the pan is screaming hot, add the olive oil and fry the sirloin strips, once seared remove onto a plate and add all the vegetables to the pan along with a splash of hot water. Steam fry the veg for 2 minutes. Now add the soy sauce, Honey and pepper flakes and stir or toss the pan until everything is evenly distributed. Finally add the cashews and sesame seeds and return the steak strips to the pan, continue to stir-fry for 1–2 more minutes and you're ready to serve.

Enjoy!

Chilli can reduce appetite and cravings. It is also has detoxifying properties due its heat.

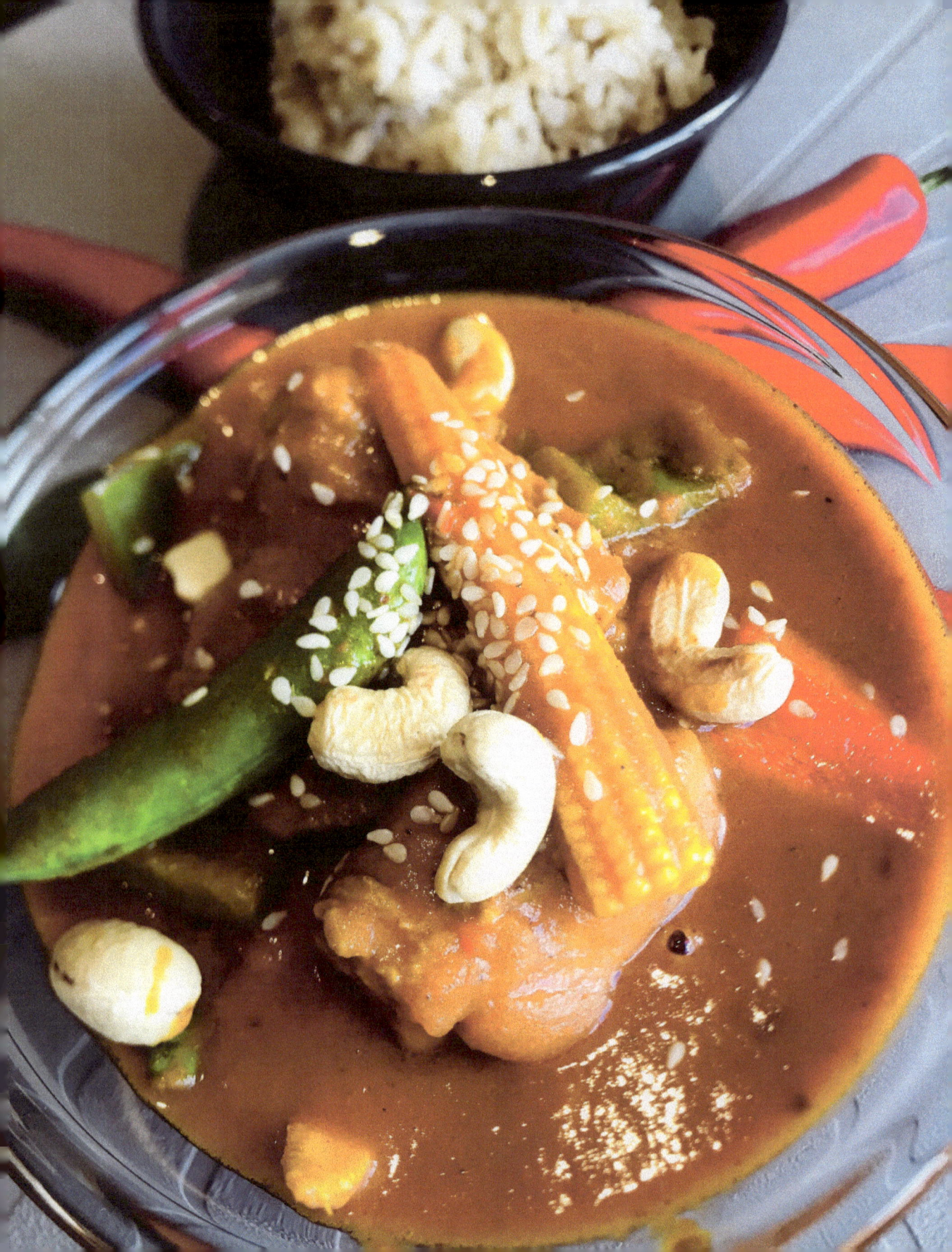

MY ULTIMATE CHICKEN CURRY

SERVES 4

8 organic chicken thighs (cut in half)

2 tbsp organic extra virgin olive oil

2 onions (peeled and roughly chopped)

2 cloves of garlic (finely chopped)

1 thumb-size piece of ginger (finely chopped)

1 red chilli (finely sliced)

1 tbsp lemongrass paste (store bought)

70 grams madras curry paste (store bought)

200 mls hot water

1 organic chicken stock cube

1 tbsp turmeric powder

400 mls coconut milk

70 grams tomato puree

250 mls tomato passata

2 tbsp good quality mango chutney

½ cup of cashew nuts (toasted)

1 tsp sesame seeds

Ground Himalayan pink salt

Freshly ground black pepper

1 green pepper (washed and cut into chunks)

1 red pepper (washed and cut into chunks)

6 baby corn (cut in half long ways)

10 sugar snap peas

Place a large stainless steel saucepan on a high heat, add the olive oil and onions and sauté for 2 minutes, add the chicken thighs and cook for 5 minutes, stirring continuously, now add the garlic, ginger, chilli, lemongrass paste and curry paste, stir well and cook for another 5 minutes. Dissolve the stock cube in the hot water and add to the pot, followed by the coconut milk, tomato puree, tomato passata and mango chutney. Bring to the boil, turn down the heat and simmer for 1 hour, stirring regularly. This will allow the sauce to thicken slightly and the chicken to tenderise. Time to stir in your crunchy vegetables, add the peppers, corn and snap peas. Finally season to taste with your salt and pepper.

Serve with wholegrain brown rice and garnish with the cashew nuts and sesame seeds.

Cashew nuts support healthy brain function and mood.

MAGIC MOUSSAKA

SERVES 6

2 tbsp organic extra virgin olive oil + more for the mash

500 grams organic grass-fed minced lamb

1 onion (finely diced)

2 carrots (peeled and finely diced)

4 ribs of celery (finely sliced)

2 cloves garlic (finely chopped)

1 tsp dried oregano

1 sprig of fresh thyme

1 sprig of fresh rosemary

1 tbsp vegetable bouillon powder

500 mls hot water

70 grams tomato puree

250 mls tomato passata

20 grams fresh curly parsley (finely chopped)

1 aubergine (finely sliced)

1 courgette (finely sliced)

2 large sweet potatoes (peeled and roughly chopped)

50 grams Parmigiano Reggiano (grated)

Ground Himalayan pink salt

Freshly ground black pepper

Place a large saucepan on a high heat, add olive oil, onions, carrot, celery and garlic and sauté for 2–3 minutes. Now add the lamb followed by all the herbs, the hot water and bouillon, stir well, making sure the lamb is well broken down with no clumps, bring to the boil and reduce the liquid by two-thirds, stirring regularly, this should take around 20-25 minutes approx.. You can remove the rosemary and thyme sprigs at this stage, then add the tomato puree and tomato passata, stir well and cook for a further 10 minutes on a medium heat. Finally season well with your salt and pepper and ¼ of the parsley.

Meanwhile place the sweet potatoes in a medium sized pot and cover with boiling water, get them on to boil. Once tender, drain well and return them to the same pot, add ¼ of the parsley and parmesan, season well with salt and pepper, and mash well.

Take a baking tray (20 cm × 26 cm × 5 cm) and lightly grease with olive oil, and start layering up your moussaka, with the sliced aubergines and courgettes, one layer of aubergine topped with the lamb sauce, followed by courgettes, then lamb sauce, repeat until all the mixture is all used, Top with the sweet potato mash, use a fork to evenly distribute the mash whilst creating little peaks at the same time.

Bake the moussaka for 40 minutes at 150 °C, use a larger tray underneath the moussaka in case of any overspill.

Lamb is rich in vitamin B12 and Folate, these nutrients are necessary for a healthy central nervous system.

TOFU SATAY WITH BROCCOLI

SERVES 2–3

1 tbsp organic extra virgin olive oil

1 onion (peeled and cut into large wedges)

2 cloves garlic (finely chopped)

1 red chilli (deseeded and finely sliced)

1 tsp ginger paste (store bought)

1 tsp lemongrass paste (store bought)

1 carrot (peeled and finely sliced)

2 ribs celery (washed and finely sliced)

1 red pepper (washed and cut up chunky)

400 mls coconut milk

1 tbsp vegetable bouillon

2 tbsp light soy sauce

2 heaped tbsp organic peanut butter

15 grams fresh coriander (roughly chopped)

280 grams organic tofu

200 grams tender stem broccoli

Place a medium stainless steel pot on a high heat, add the olive oil, followed by the onion, garlic, chilli, ginger paste, lemongrass paste, carrot, celery and pepper, cook and stir for 5 minutes. Add the coconut milk, vegetable bouillon, soy sauce and peanut butter, stir well and bring to the boil, turn the heat down to a simmer and add the tofu and coriander, continue to simmer for 10 minutes to allow the tofu to take on the flavour of the sauce.

Meanwhile plunge your broccoli into a pot of boiling salted water for 2 minutes and you're ready to serve.

Enjoy!

Tofu is a good source of tryptophan, which helps in stress management and supports better sleep.

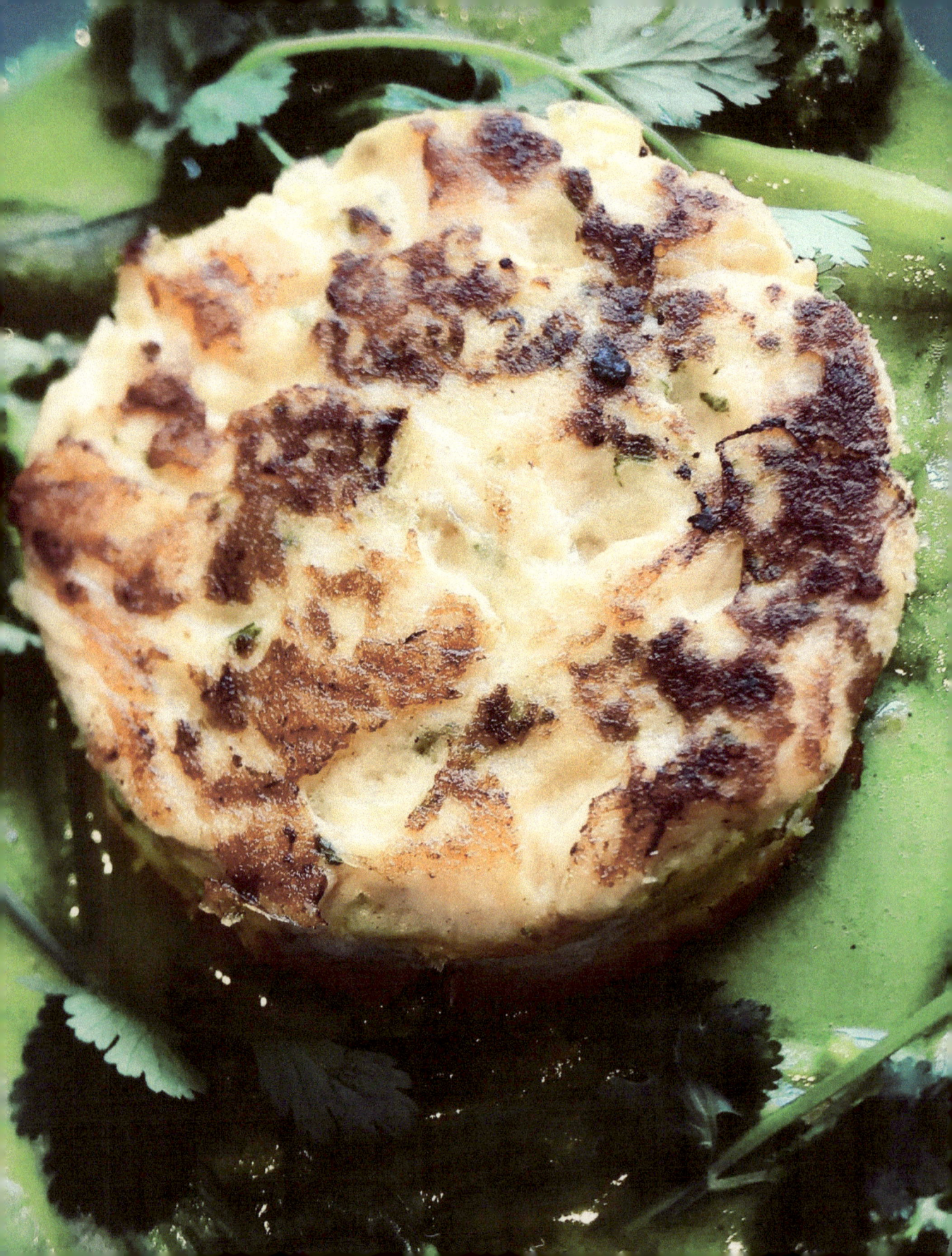

THAI GREEN CURRY WITH SALMON FISHCAKE AND COCONUT QUINOA

SERVES 2

FOR THE QUINOA

½ cup quinoa

400 mls coconut milk

1 tsp vegetable bouillon powder

Place all ingredients in a small pot and bring to the boil, simmer for 10–12 minutes or until the quinoa has absorbed all the liquid, remove from the heat and put a lid on the pot, leave to the side for 15 minutes and your done with this.

FOR THE CURRY

Sauce;

400 mls coconut milk

30 grams fresh coriander

4 spring onions

½ green pepper

1 thumb sized piece of ginger

2 cloves garlic

1 green chilli

1 tsp lemongrass paste

1 tsp vegetable bouillon powder

Veg;

1 pak choi

½ green pepper (cut into chunks)

5 snap peas

5 mange tout

3 stems of broccoli

Place all the sauce ingredients into the nutribullet and blitz for 1 minute, then pour into a medium sized pot, bring to the boil, add the veg and season well with ground Himalayan pink salt and freshly ground black pepper. Second stage done!

SALMON FISHCAKE

400 grams of fresh salmon (belly meat, if you can get it)

2 spring onions (finely chopped)

1 tsp lemongrass paste

1 organic egg

Place half of the salmon into a food processor with the spring onions, lemongrass paste and egg. Season well with salt and pepper and blitz to form a thick mousse. Cut the remaining salmon into small chunks and mix with the mousse in a large bowl. Place a non-stick frying pan on a high heat and put 2 lightly greased stainless steel 9 cm cooking rings in the pan, drizzle a little olive oil into each ring and divide the salmon mixture between the 2 rings, pressing down with a spoon. Fry for 2 minutes each side, finish the cooking in a hot oven (200 °C) for 15 minutes approx. until piping hot all the way through. Use a knife to free the cakes from the rings and serve with the sauce and quinoa. BOOM!

Coriander is a fantastic chelating herb, it contains detoxifying, antibacterial and immune enhancing oils. It can help remove heavy metals from the body.

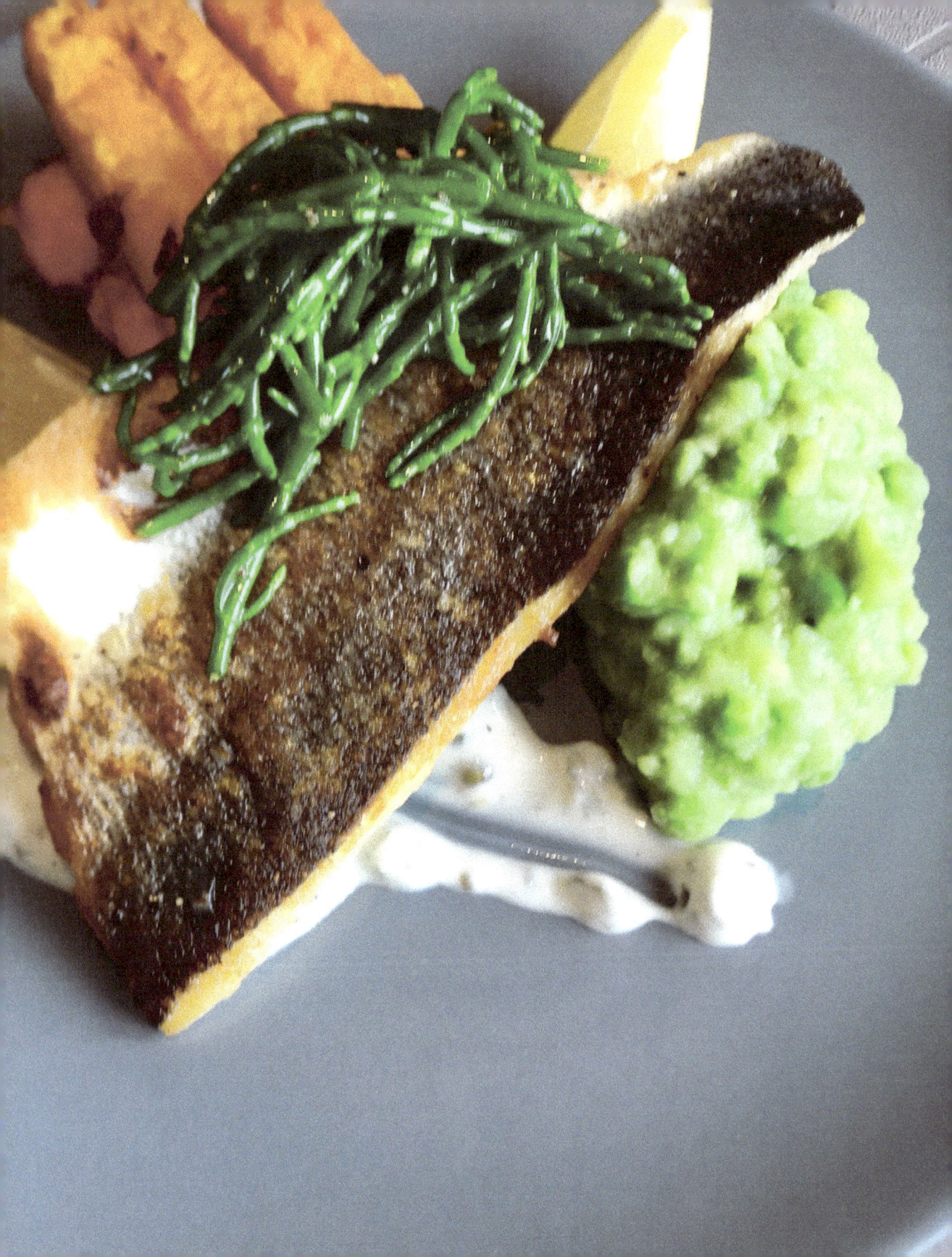

FISH 'N' CHIPS

SERVES 2

Organic extra virgin olive oil

2 fresh seabass fillets (boneless and descaled)

1 large sweet potato (peeled and cut into chunky chips)

50 grams samphire

1 lemon (cut into wedges)

Place the chips in the acti-fry with 1 tbsp olive oil and season with pink salt, set the timer for 20 minutes for perfect chips (alternatively brush with olive oil and bake in a hot oven, 200 °C, for 20 minutes).

FOR THE TARTARE SAUCE

150 grams organic bio live yoghurt

1 tbsp capers (finely chopped)

5 cocktail gherkins (finely chopped)

juice from 1 lemon wedge

Mix together the yoghurt, capers, gherkins and lemon juice and season well with ground Himalayan pink salt and freshly ground black pepper.

FOR THE MUSHY PEAS

1 300 gram can of mushy peas

1 handful of frozen garden peas

1 tbsp apple cider vinegar (with the mother)

Place the 2 types of peas in a small pot and warm through on a gentle heat, add the vinegar and season well with your salt and pepper.

FOR THE FISH

Place a large non-stick frying pan on a high heat, rub the seabass fillets with a little olive oil and season well with your salt and pepper. Gently place the fillets skin side down in the pan and fry for 3–4 minutes, check for a golden skin, then turn over and finish cooking for 2 minutes, remove from the pan and rest on a plate for 1 minute. Place the samphire in the same pan with a splash of water and steam fry for 1–2 minutes until just tender.

Assemble all the elements on your serving plates, squeeze your lemon wedge over the fish, and enjoy.

Bio live yoghurt – live cultures in yoghurt can improve the microflora in the gut.

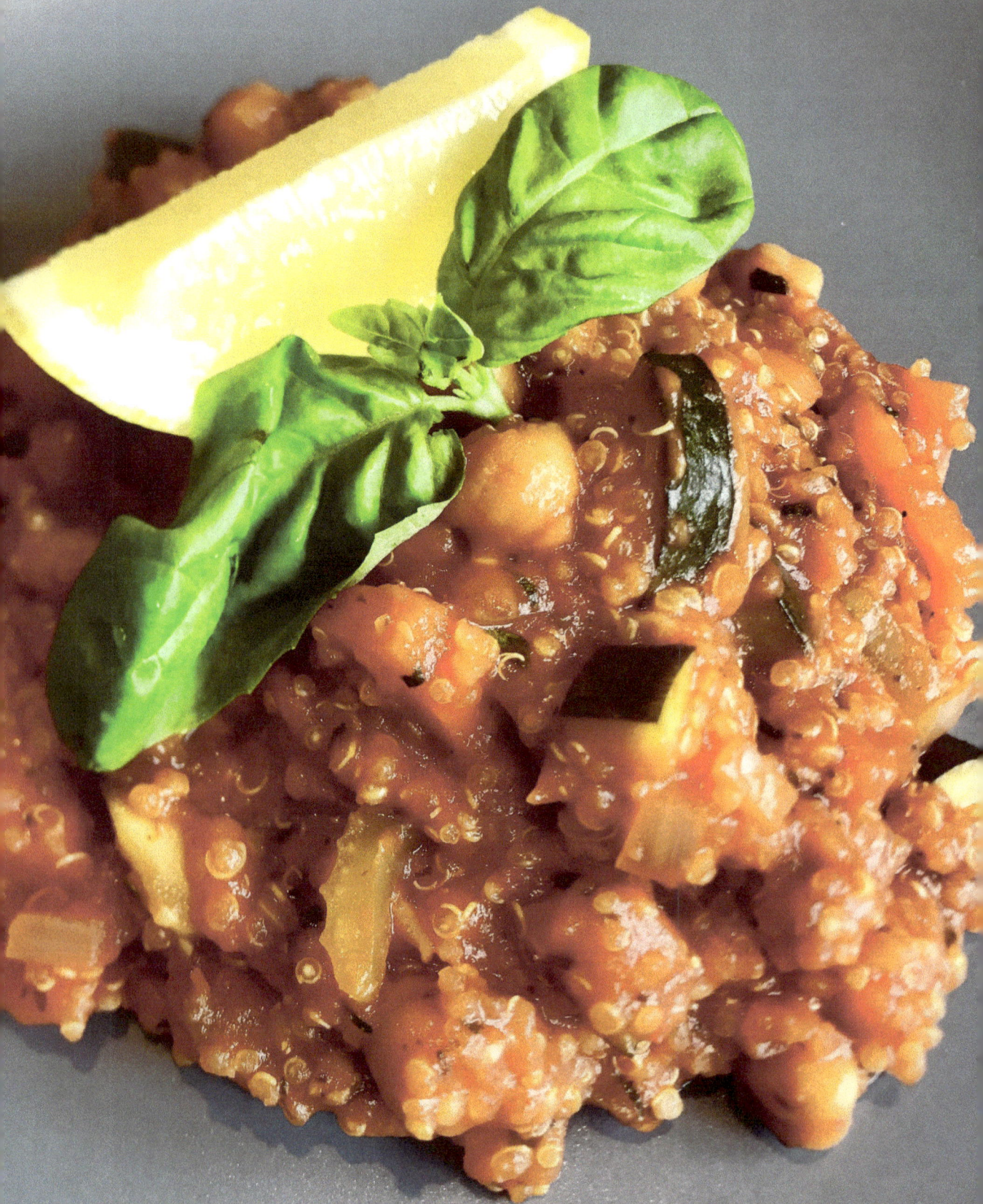

QUINOA CHILLI CON VEGETALI

SERVES 3–4

1 tbsp organic extra virgin olive oil

1 onion (peeled and roughly chopped)

2 cloves garlic (finely chopped)

2 ribs celery (finely sliced)

1 carrot (peeled and diced)

1 courgette (washed and cut into small chunks)

1 red pepper (washed and cut up chunky)

1 tbsp dried oregano

1 tbsp piri piri spice

1 tbsp vegetable bouillon powder

130 grams of drained canned chickpeas

½ cup quinoa

1 cup hot water

70 grams tomato puree

200 mls tomato passata

10 fresh basil leaves (finely chopped)

Juice from half lemon

1 tbsp sriracha chilli sauce

Place a large stainless steel pot on a medium heat, add the olive oil, followed by the onions, garlic, celery, carrot, courgette, pepper, oregano and piri piri spice, cook for 5 minutes stirring continuously. Now add the vegetable bouillon, chickpeas, quinoa, hot water, tomato puree and tomato passata. Stir thoroughly ensuring everything is evenly distributed, turn the heat down, put a lid on and cook for 30 minutes stirring occasionally. Finish with the chopped basil, lemon juice and sriracha sauce, stirring thoroughly again before serving.

Enjoy!

Oregano is antibacterial and protects against free radical damage.

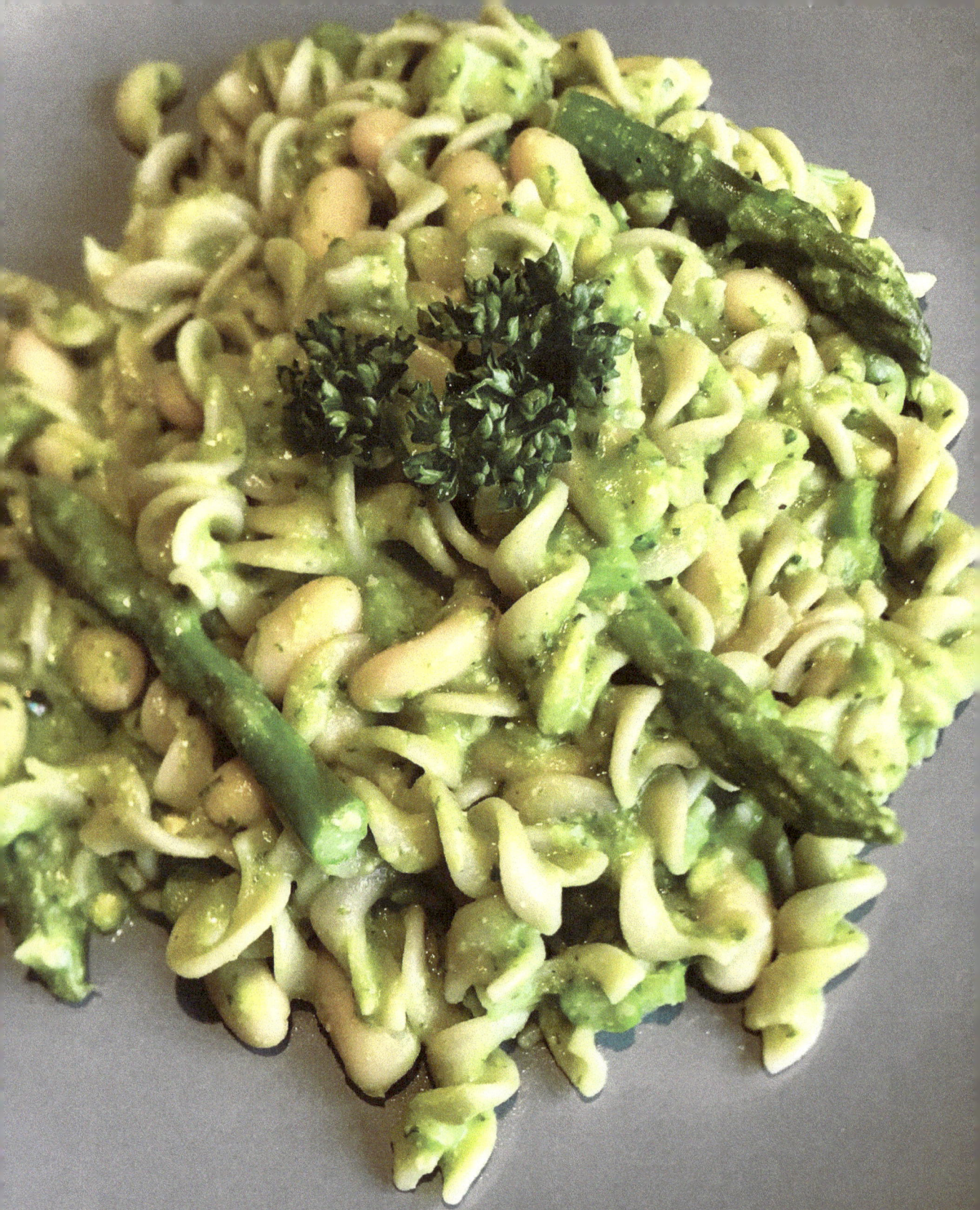

PASTA PRIMAVERA VERDI

SERVES 2–3

250 grams brown rice pasta

150 grams asparagus (woody end removed, finely chopped, leave spears intact)

1 400 ml can cannellini beans (drained and rinsed)

FOR THE AVOCADO PESTO

1 ripe avocado (stone and skin removed)

1 handful of baby spinach

½ cup toasted cashew nuts

2 cloves garlic

15 grams fresh parsley (stems removed and finely chopped)

Juice of ½ lemon

4 tbsp organic extra virgin olive oil

Ground Himalayan pink salt

Freshly ground black pepper

Cook the pasta according to pack instructions in a large pot of boiling salted water for about 9–10 minutes, meanwhile make the pesto.

Place the avocado, spinach, nuts, garlic, parsley, lemon juice and olive oil into a food processer and season well with your salt and pepper. Blitz until relatively smooth, with some texture remaining.

When the pasta is almost cooked (around 7–8 minutes) add the asparagus and beans to the pasta pot and boil for another 2 minutes. This way the pasta, asparagus and beans are all ready at the same time. Drain off the pasta, but leave behind a good ½ cup approx. of the pasta water in the pot (this helps create your sauce).

Add the pesto to the pasta pot and stir well and you're ready to serve.

Spinach is high in vitamin K which is important for maintaining healthy bones, it also contains more than a dozen different antioxidant compounds that help fight inflammation.

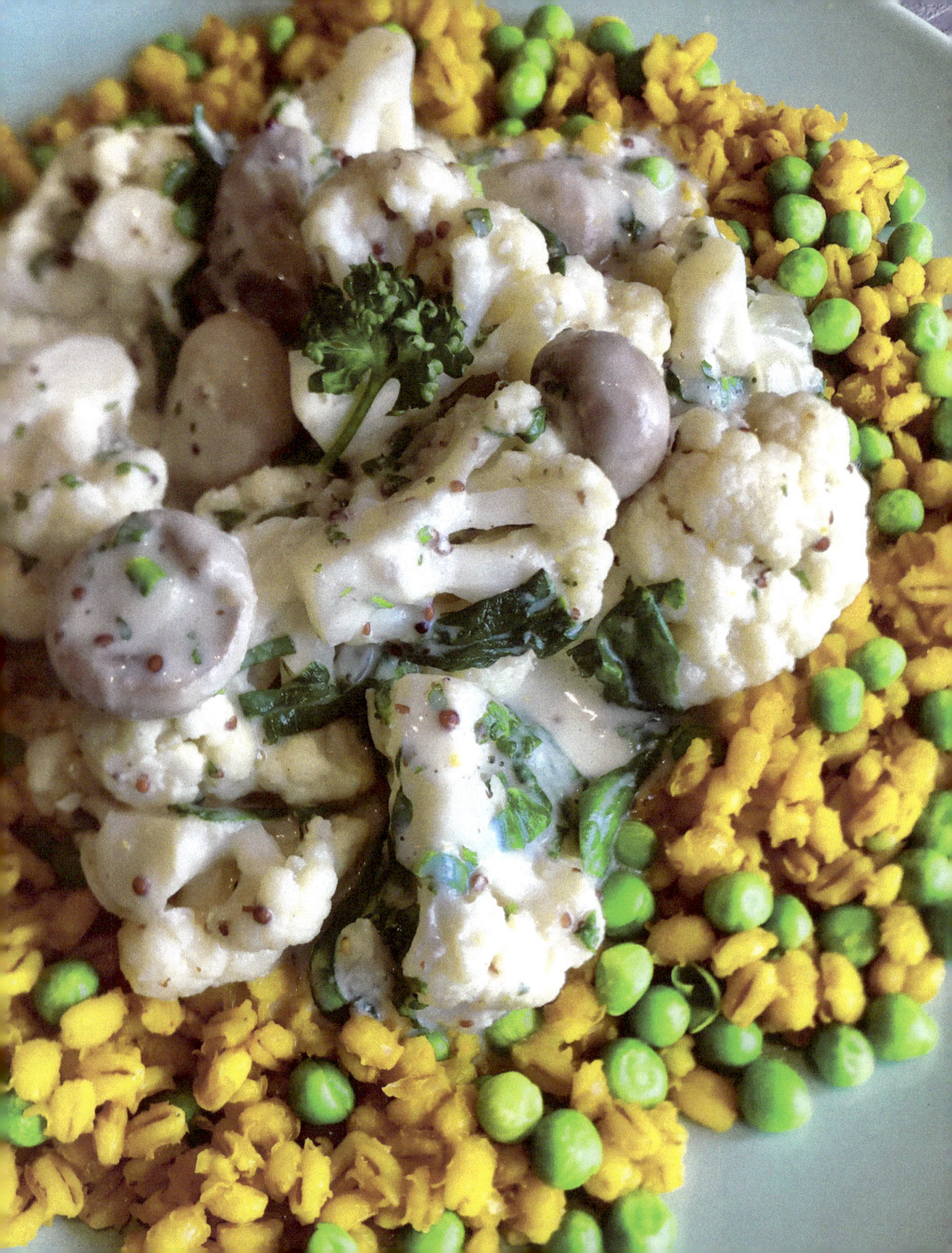

CAULIFLOWER FRICASSEE WITH PEAS & BARLEY

SERVES 2

FOR THE PEAS AND BARLEY

½ cup pearl barley (soaked in water overnight) (contains gluten)

1 tbsp turmeric powder

½ cup frozen peas

Cook the barley in a medium size pot with the turmeric and plenty of boiling salted water for 50–60 minutes (you will need to top up the boiling water several times) or until very tender, then add the peas to the pot for 1 minute to warm through, then drain and rinse with a full kettle of boiling water (this gets rid of a lot of glutenous starch).

FOR THE FRICASSEE

1 tbsp organic extra virgin olive oil

½ onion (finely chopped)

100 grams button mushrooms (cleaned)

2 cloves garlic (finely chopped)

2 sprigs thyme

250 mls oat cream

1 tbsp vegetable bouillon powder

1 tbsp wholegrain mustard

400 grams cauliflower florets

1 handful baby spinach (finely chopped)

10 grams fresh parsley (stems removed and finely chopped)

freshly ground black pepper

In a large pot fry the onions, mushrooms garlic and thyme with the olive oil for 5 minutes on a medium heat, stirring continuously, add the oat cream, bouillon and mustard and bring to the boil. Now add the cauliflower, stir well, put a lid on and cook for 6–7 minutes on a medium heat, until the cauliflower is just tender with a little bite. Finally add the spinach and parsley, season well with black pepper.

Serve the fricassee with the peas and barley.

Freshly ground black pepper stimulates appetite and aids digestion.

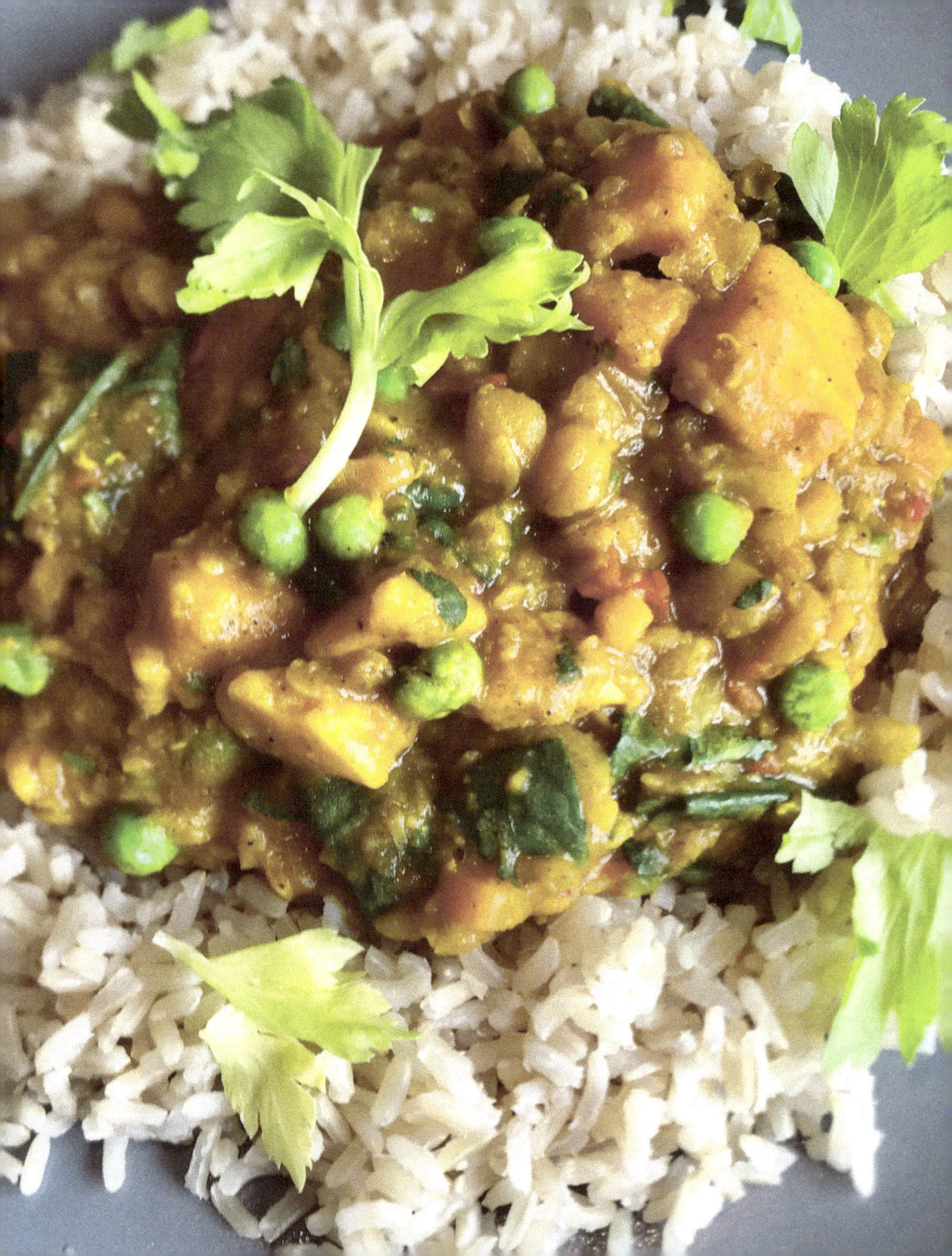

SWEET POTATO AND SPINACH DAHL

SERVES 2–3

1 tbsp organic extra virgin olive oil

½ onion (finely chopped)

1 carrot (peeled and finely diced)

2 ribs celery (washed and finely sliced)

1 red chilli (deseeded and finely chopped)

1 thumb-size piece of ginger (peeled and finely chopped)

2 cloves garlic (finely chopped)

70 grams madras curry paste (store bought)

½ cup yellow lentils

500 mls hot water

1 tbsp vegetable bouillon powder

½ cup red lentils

1 large sweet potato (peeled and cut into chunks)

250 mls hot water

½ cup frozen peas

1 handful baby spinach

10 grams chopped coriander

Cooked wholegrain brown rice

To a large pot, add the olive oil, followed by the onion, carrot, celery, chilli, ginger and garlic and sauté for 5 minutes, stirring continuously on a medium heat, then add the yellow lentils, the 500 mls of hot water and the bouillon. Stir well and simmer for 10 minutes. Now add the red lentils, sweet potato and the remaining 250 mls of hot water, stir well, turn the heat down low and simmer for 50 minutes, or until all the lentils and sweet potato are well cooked and tender. Finally add the peas, spinach and coriander, stir well and cook for a further 2–3 minutes.

Serve up with wholegrain brown rice.

Enjoy!

Lentils are rich in vitamin B1 (thiamine) which helps to regulate the nervous system.

EXAMPLE WEEKLY MEAL PLANNER

	MON	TUE	WED	THU	FRI	SAT	SUN
Rise							
B/Fast							
Snack							
Lunch							
Snack							
Dinner							

MY WEEKLY MEAL PLANNER

	MON	TUE	WED	THU	FRI	SAT	SUN
Rise							
B/Fast							
Snack							
Lunch							
Snack							
Dinner							

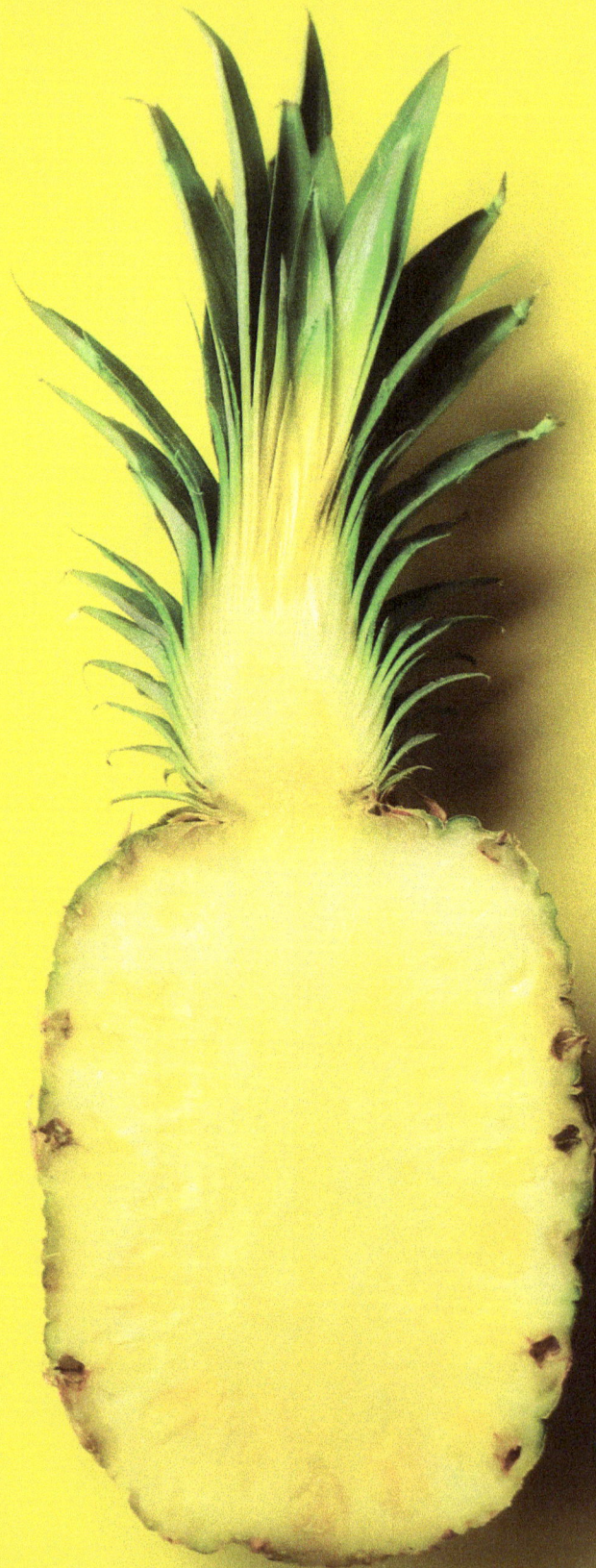

ACKNOWLEDGEMENTS

I would like to thank Danny O Rawe (CNM Nutrition lecturer & Belfast Herbalist) for empowering me with great knowledge, and for his support and encouragement when I told him I was going to do this book. I would also like to thank Nicola Cantley (CNM Clinical Supervisor, Nutrition Lecturer & Nutritional Therapist), because she inspired me to structure the book in such a way, dictated by what we as nutritionists in clinic were giving as advice to our clients. Ultimately this book was exactly the tool that we needed to motivate people (but didn't have) in order for clients to make better food choices, and so I constructed and collated these recipes and tips, because I believe there is nothing like this on the market.

Finally I would like to extend my gratitude to Gareth and the team at Authoright, who really brought this book to life. I'm looking forward to starting on my second book and working with Authoright once again.

DISCLAIMER

Whilst every effort has been made to ensure the information in this book, is complete and accurate, the suggestions made are not intended as a substitute for individual medical advice. Always consult your doctor before changing your diet!

www.ingramcontent.com/pod-product-compliance
Lightning Source LLC
Chambersburg PA
CBHW041017280326
41926CB00094B/4660